the
metabolic
clock

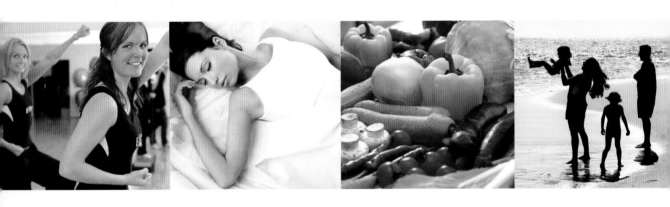

the
metabolic
clock

METABOLISE

MOMENTUM

10am · 2pm

ENERGISE

6am · 6pm

CREATE

RELAX

2am · REJUVENATE · 10pm

speed up your metabolism and lose weight easily

Julie Rennie

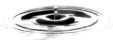

ROCKPOOL
PUBLISHING

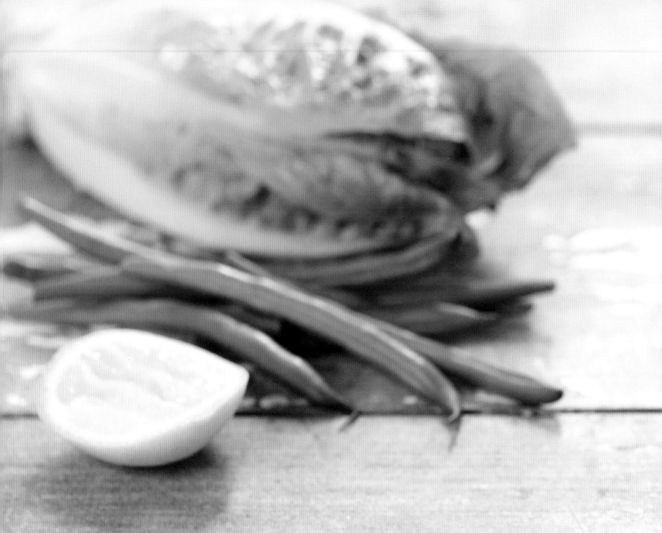

A Rockpool book
Published by Rockpool Publishing
24 Constitution Road, Dulwich Hill,
NSW 2203, Australia

www.rockpoolpublishing.com.au

First published in 2011

Printed by Everbest, China
10 9 8 7 6 5 4 3 2

National Library of Australia
Cataloguing-in-Publication entry

Rennie, Julie.

The metabolic clock ; speed up your metabolism
and lose weight easily / Julie Rennie.

1st ed.

9781921295317 (pbk.)

Includes index.
Reducing diets.
Reducing exercises.

613.25

Edited by Jody Lee and Megan Drinan
Cover and internal design by Stan Lamond
Food Photographer: Brent Parker Jones
Food Stylist: Lee Blaylock
Food Stylist assistants: Julie Rennie, Gareth Thomas

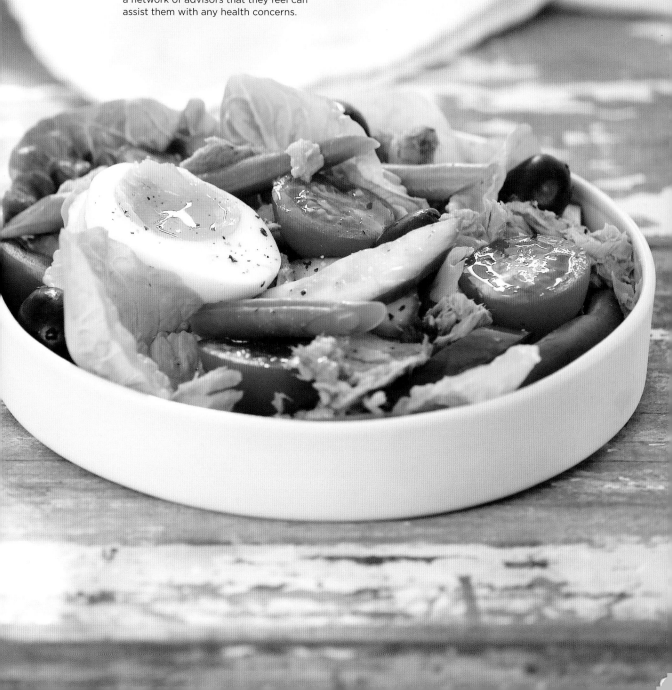

Contents

A message from the author   8

Introduction   10

Step 1

How to speed up your metabolism to burn body fat and create more energy   13

Chapter 1   The Metabolic Clock   17

Chapter 2   Balancing your metabolic clock   21

Chapter 3   Revitalise your digestive system   35

Chapter 4   Move your body to feel good about yourself   45

Chapter 5   Nourishment strategies for maximum energy   51

Step 2

How to create the motivation to attain your weight loss and wellness goals   61

Chapter 6   Start thinking like a healthy person   62

Chapter 7   Create impassioned thinking   64

Chapter 8   Mind sweep to clear out your disempowering thoughts   68

Chapter 9   Create an 'I can attitude' – changing bad habits with three empowering strategies   73

Chapter 10   Believe everything is possible   76

Chapter 11   Visualize your success   79

Step 3

How to get started and gain momentum 81

Chapter 12   Plan for success 82

Chapter 13   Clean out your cupboards 84

Chapter 14   Inspire yourself to achieve with a 21-Day Lifestyle Challenge 86

Chapter 15   Getting your Metabolic Clock kitchen organized and planning your meals 90

Chapter 16   Kitchen helpers 94

The Metabolic Clock recipes 103

Morning juice 104

Breakfast 106

Mid-morning fruit 116

Midday meal 118

Mid-afternoon snacks 131

Evening meal 134

Sweet treats and tea 152

Eating out 159

Putting *The Metabolic Clock* meal plans into action 160

How to use the weekly meal plans 161

Warm weather menu plans 162

Cold weather menu plans 165

A simple formula for sustainable weight loss 168

The Metabolic Clock wrap-up 169

Bibliography 170

Index 171

A message from the author

As I approached middle age it seemed every year I was slowly gaining more weight. I justified this weight gain and my lack of vitality as part of the ageing process. I would come home from a busy day at work feeling sorry for myself and too tired to cook dinner. I wasn't organized enough to have any healthy food in the house and decided that a glass of wine and some chocolate would make me feel better. This had become a very common lifestyle choice that I was making – and it was also making me feel very guilty.

My thoughts went like this: 'I need to be healthier. Why can't I get motivated to diet? I must stop drinking so much alcohol. I should be exercising. Why can't I get organized? Why am I feeling so bloated and sluggish?' And so it went on. I felt frustrated with myself and knew that as soon as my head hit the pillow my negative thoughts would take over, spiralling me into a restless night of self-judgment.

After yet another sleepless night I thought, 'I don't need another diet, I need a lifestyle that works for me.' Diets only work when you are on them and I did *not* want to be on a diet for the rest of my life. This decision led me to amazing discoveries about my health and wellbeing. At the same time I realized that my lack of motivation came from negative thoughts about myself. So the first thing I decided to do was to learn how to create empowering self-talk, which has become my motivation rocket fuel.

As I started on my journey of self-discovery and empowerment I discovered Ayurveda; an ancient system of medicine and healing that creates harmony between mind, body and the forces of nature. I then applied the principles of this ancient wisdom to achieve balance in my hectic Western lifestyle. And to my surprise, I lost weight without even trying. Quite by accident, I had discovered how to speed up my metabolism and burn off body fat easily.

Delving deeper, I looked into the scientific research that verified this ancient wisdom. In doing so, I discovered that our bodies have natural cycles that control and manage appetite, energy, mood and sleep, called circadian rhythms. When these are out of balance, nothing feels right – but when they are in balance, we are at our best.

Paying attention to circadian rhythms really suited my lifestyle *and* me. I didn't have time to count calories; I had no energy to exercise; and I loved my food too much to drink shakes or go on a diet. Simply adapting my lifestyle to a more natural cycle, I found I had more energy and felt like exercising. I also needed less sleep, which meant I had more time to do the things I enjoyed in life.

This was the beginning of *The Metabolic Clock*.

My partner was on a diet and eating pre-packaged, portion-controlled meals. He was losing weight – but it was a slow process – and he was miserable because he wasn't enjoying the food.

One night we sat down to dinner. I had a big plate of food and he looked at his uninspiring portion-controlled meal. He kept looking at my plate and he said, 'I don't get it. You eat twice as much as me *and* you eat a piece of chocolate every day. Worse, you hardly exercise. I am sweating it out at the gym six days a week and starving myself on this tasteless food and you are losing weight quicker than me. What's your secret?'

My secret is balance. I had made lifestyle changes that reset my body clock and tuned it into nature's rhythms. I had also learned what to eat and when to speed up my metabolism – this boosted my energy and I lost weight without being on a diet.

From that moment, my partner decided to use the simple weight loss and wellness secrets of the Metabolic Clock. To his surprise, he shed 22 kilos (48lbs) of body fat easily and started to enjoy feeling more energized, too.

The lifestyle changes that I made were so simple and very natural. It's funny that we don't notice that we are well, only when we are unwell. That's because being a healthy weight and feeling energized *is* our natural state: the state your body is most comfortable with. When you make healthy changes towards how you take care of yourself, your body will reward you with a wellspring of energy and you will easily and comfortably lose weight.

After a few years of experiencing renewed health and wellbeing, I decided to return to competitive track running, which I had not done for 14 years. I had all the energy I needed to do the training, but had not anticipated that my ageing muscles would take some time to catch up.

In my enthusiasm to compete, I tore a calf muscle while running and fell, breaking my wrist. My injuries meant that I could not exercise for eight weeks. During this time, I focused solely on the lifestyle strategies of *The Metabolic Clock* and without exercising at all, I still lost weight. If you are a person who absolutely does not like to raise a sweat, then this system will still work for you.

When some mothers at my son's school asked me what I was doing to have so much energy, I decided to give my time and this powerful information for free. I created a pilot program and began sharing it with small groups of people. So many achieved amazing weight loss and enjoyed an increase in energy levels that it wasn't long before I was asked to speak at corporate events about the Metabolic Clock and how it can be used to achieve work–life balance. Then celebrities and Olympic athletes wanted to use the Metabolic Clock to balance their busy lifestyles, too.

When you align yourself with the natural energy cycles of the Metabolic Clock, you will feel more empowered to make healthy lifestyle changes. Once you learn the Metabolic Clock lifestyle for easy, sustainable weight loss, you will have it for life! You won't need to spend any more money on pre-packaged, portion-controlled diet food, weight-loss products or diet shakes. The Metabolic Clock will give you a lifetime of health and wellbeing. It's a blueprint for great health and vitality. You might occasionally step out of this lifestyle, but I guarantee you will go right back to it because you will want to retain the feeling of wellbeing that this lifestyle will give you.

If you are a busy person who wants to know how to be healthy and live with more balance, then you will love the simplicity of the Metabolic Clock. I have shared this information with thousands of people, either personally or at seminars and events, with amazing results. Try it for yourself.

How else will you know it works unless you try it?

Julie Rennie

Introduction

Welcome to *The Metabolic Clock*. It is full of simple, natural, weight-loss strategies that will get you started on your journey to achieving a healthy, slim body.

Why follow *The Metabolic Clock*?

Diets only work for the short time you are on them, and who wants to be on a diet for the rest of their life anyway? You can count calories to lose weight, but you may only be making an unhealthy diet smaller.

You can cut out all the carbohydrates and fats from your diet and always feel that you are hungry and missing something. Or you can see a health professional who gives you a long list of foods that you are not allowed to eat and look in your fridge and cupboard and think, 'What am I going to eat?'

You can purchase pre-packaged, portion-controlled meals and lose weight while you diet. Then when you stop eating these meals, you may put all the weight back on plus, sometimes more.

You can be taken in by fad diets and the promises of quick weight loss products and unbalance your metabolism, leaving you feeling sluggish.

Or, you can use the strategies of *The Metabolic Clock* to create a balanced approach to losing weight and being healthy that lasts a lifetime.

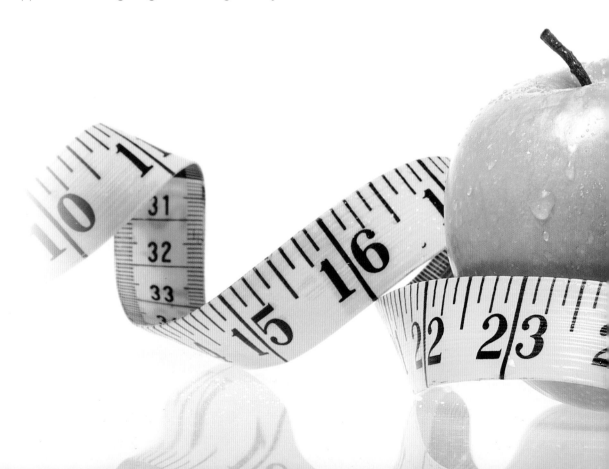

The Metabolic Clock action plan

By reading this book, you will be able to create an action plan to achieve a healthy, slim body. You will:

- be inspired to create your own wellness goals and understand the compelling reasons to attain them
- learn how to create a balanced daily routine and understand why it is so important to your overall health
- learn how to implement simple strategies that will speed up your metabolism; boost your energy; and make it easy to burn body fat without being on a diet
- implement six daily practices that will revitalise your digestive system
- find the motivation to exercise because you will understand the value of moving your body as a way to feel good about yourself
- use tools that will help you overcome emotional eating and build your motivation to achieve your goals
- have a formula to help you clean out your cupboards so that you can create a clean foundation for creating your compelling new future
- start a 21-Day Lifestyle Challenge to create a healthy and balanced daily routine
- be motivated to get your kitchen organized with healthy food.

You've taken the step that will help you to discover what you can do to get your metabolism moving. Not only will you lose weight and gain health, but you won't feel like you are missing out on the good things in life.

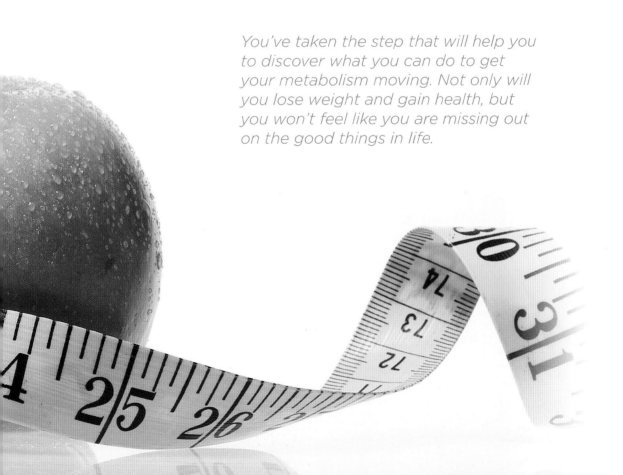

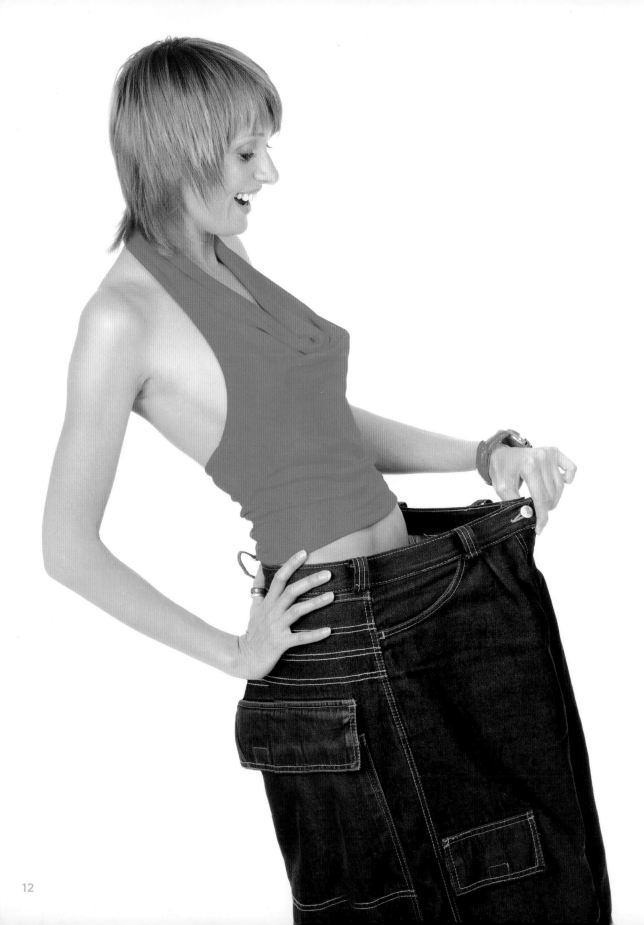

Step 1

How to speed up your metabolism to burn body fat and create more energy

'The key to keeping your balance is knowing when you've lost it.'

When your metabolic clock is in balance with nature's rhythms, your metabolism speeds up, you burn body fat easily, you have lots of energy, you sleep well and you naturally feel balanced and healthy. In this section you will learn what to eat, when to eat and what activities are best suited throughout the day, according to your natural energy cycles.

Creating compelling reasons to change your lifestyle

'The bigger the why, the easier the how' – Jim Rohn

To get started, you will need to decide why you would like to be healthy and enjoy a slim, comfortable body. Why is this important to you? Here are some examples to get you started.
- Summer is approaching and I want to look good in a bathing suit.
- I have an important function coming up and would like to fit into a smaller dress size.
- I am in a new relationship.
- I would like to get into shape to attract a new partner.
- My doctor has warned me about my health.
- I would like to feel better and have more energy.
- I would like to be more active and play more with my kids.
- I have booked a holiday and want to get fit for it.
- I would like to be fit enough to play a sport.

It's really important to know why this wellness journey is important to you. It doesn't matter what other people think; they don't know *your* dreams and goals. You may like to buy a journal so that you can write down your thoughts and any inspirations that you discover as you journey towards your weight-loss and wellness goals.

Your personal reasons will get you through any setbacks or obstacles you may experience along the way. Remember to keep reminding yourself of the outcome you would like to reach and why it's important to you.

Think of yourself as an athlete. All great athletes had to start somewhere and they all experience setbacks and plateaus along the way. What keeps them focused and training is that they continually think of the outcome of winning. Without this they would not be motivated to train in the rain, hail or heat waves. Without personal reasons, it would be easy to give up when the going gets tough.

Creating your wellness goals

Next, take a few moments to create your wellness goals. These differ from your compelling reasons to change your lifestyle. They are specific things that you would like to achieve, for example:

- lower my cholesterol
- lose 5 kilos (11 lbs)
- give up smoking
- run a 10 km (6 mile) fun run
- join a gym and train three times a week
- get six-pack abs
- learn how to cook healthy food
- lower my blood pressure
- create a healthy daily routine.

First get your goals clear in your mind – there is no right or wrong answer, just think about things that are relevant or have meaning to you and your situation. When you have created wellness goals in your mind, write them down in your journal.

Keep your compelling reasons and wellness goals in a place where you can see them every day.

Write your compelling reasons and wellness goals down on a sheet of paper and place them on the refrigerator door, or stick them on the bathroom mirror. Keep looking at them so that they are always at the front of your mind, not buried under the negative thinking that so often clutters our minds. If you have a moment where you are feeling unmotivated, choose to replace these thoughts with ones of achieving your goals and all the reasons why this is important to you. Now that you've decided what your wellness goals are, take a moment to fill out the following questionnaire to identify any obstacles.

What is optimal wellness for you?

_____

_____

_____

What is holding you back from creating optimal wellness?

- ☐ Lack of motivation
- ☐ Not knowing how
- ☐ Because of past failures
- ☐ Lack of information
- ☐ Not enough time
- ☐ Believe that it is all too hard

- ☐ Have not made the decision to change
- ☐ Do not believe that it is possible
- ☐ Have no support structure
- ☐ Have not made the commitment
- ☐ Don't have enough money
- ☐ Too tired and have no energy

Are you currently experiencing?

- ☐ Illness or ailment
- ☐ Loss of someone close
- ☐ Illness of someone close
- ☐ Unresolved pain from the past
- ☐ Feelings of failure
- ☐ Depression or anxiety
- ☐ A fear of getting old
- ☐ Stresses in life
- ☐ Putting off decisions

- ☐ Feelings of anger
- ☐ Relationship issues
- ☐ Financial pressures
- ☐ Family issues
- ☐ Fear of the future
- ☐ Issues from the past
- ☐ Life is outside of my control
- ☐ Feel isolated
- ☐ Lack happiness and joy

Do you emotionally eat or take stimulants when?

- ☐ Stressed or upset
- ☐ Bored or lonely
- ☐ Angry
- ☐ Escaping from something
- ☐ Feeling unfulfilled

- ☐ Trying to relax
- ☐ Feeling destructive
- ☐ Looking for a lift
- ☐ Not feeling worthy or deserving
- ☐ In emotional pain

Current eating habits

- ☐ Do you eat your food quickly?
- ☐ Do you eat without chewing?
- ☐ When you eat, is your mind on something else?
- ☐ Do you eat on the run?

- ☐ Do you regularly skip meals?
- ☐ Do you eat when you are anxious or stressed?
- ☐ Do you experience indigestion?
- ☐ Do you eat breakfast every day?

Be patient with yourself.

Oh, and there is one more thing. Be patient with yourself. This is not a diet. These healthy practices are a lifelong approach to your health and wellbeing so you don't need to be in a hurry. Just like an athlete, it's the persistence of doing these practices that will bring you balance and sustainable weight loss.

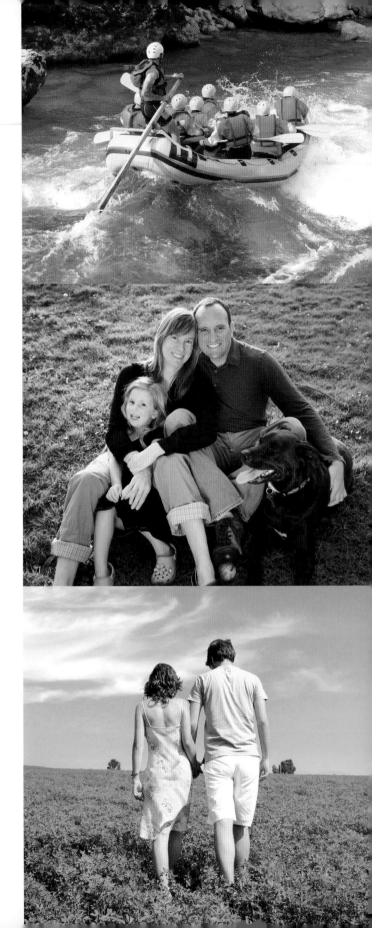

Chapter 1

The metabolic clock

What is metabolism?

The metabolism is the engine room of your body: it is the process that keeps life going. This engine room converts raw materials into fuel which is the energy your body uses to function. It also provides the resources to repair damaged tissue and rid the body of toxins. Your digestive system is literally the beginning and end of all the body's processes. It processes the food you eat, then absorbs the nutrients through a large network of tiny blood vessels, eliminating what isn't needed. Running parallel with these blood vessels is 70 per cent of your body's immune system. The immune system is your body's first line of defence from invaders such as harmful bacteria, viruses and poisonous substances.

Your digestive system is full of nerve endings. It has as many nerve endings as the spine. This is significant because what you are thinking affects how you are feeling. What you think sends messages via the central nervous system. The next time you feel anxious or nervous stop for a moment and observe your gut. Do you have butterflies in your stomach or do you feel tense from feeling nervous? Your feelings have an impact on the efficiency of your digestive system.

The digestive tract operates like a muscle. It contracts and releases; this is how food is passed through it. When you are stressed you contract these muscles but don't release them and this stops the processing of the food. On the other hand, if you are relaxed and happy this process happens quite naturally and your digestive system gets moving. The next time you feel inspired and happy notice how this affects your metabolism. Empowering thoughts energise you through your metabolism.

With all these important duties it should be no surprise that if your digestive system isn't working efficiently you'll feel sluggish, gain weight easily, lack motivation and be more susceptible to illness.

Aligning your metabolism with nature's cycles

Nature is made up of rhythms or cycles: there is sunrise, sunset, the four seasons and the 24-hour rotation of the earth. Scientific research has revealed that our bodies also have natural cycles that control and manage appetite, energy, mood and sleep. These are called circadian rhythms, also known as your body clock or metabolic clock.

When your body is in sync with nature's rhythms, your body clock or metabolic clock will respond with a balanced dose of hormones. This triggers our daily activities. When functioning properly, your body clock will respond to the light of a new day by triggering the production of cortisol, serotonin and other hormones. This wakes you up and gets you going. When the sun goes down, the body clock gets another cue and responds to dusk. It produces another hormone called melatonin, which prepares us for restful sleep.

Nature, and its 24-hour cycle of day and night, has given us a template that anticipates what we need in order to be balanced and healthy. When our body clock or metabolic clock is in sync with nature we sleep well, we eat in a more balanced way and we have lots of energy.

When we are in balance we are at our best.

However, modern living and lifestyle patterns have dramatically altered our ability to respond to nature's cues. For example, many people no longer get enough daylight or are exposed to too much unnatural light at night. This has had a dramatic effect on our hormone production.

When our body clock or metabolic clock is out of balance with nature's cycles, nothing seems to feel right. This is because the hormones, chemicals and neurotransmitters that determine our mood, how we sleep and our appetite get out of balance.

What is your metabolic clock?

The metabolic clock is your internal body clock, which cues you to be in balance with nature's rhythms so that you have the right energy at the right time to perform the functions of your daily life comfortably and easily. In recognizing this natural 24-hour cycle you can maximise your metabolism for peak digestion, burn body fat more easily and have more energy for daily living. A balanced metabolic clock will have you feeling inspired, energized and empowered.

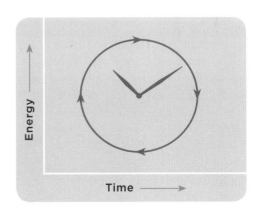

Constant dieting disrupts the metabolic clock

Your body's metabolic clock is finely balanced and automatically responds to nature's daily cycles. Anything that disrupts your metabolic clock will put you and your system out of kilter, creating all manner of imbalances.

For example, when you wake up, your metabolic clock signals to you that it's hungry and needs food to fuel it. If you are dieting, by skipping a meal or cutting back on food to save on calories, you override this natural signal. When your metabolic clock registers that no food is available, your body responds by slowing down the metabolism to save on fuel. Slowing down the metabolism is a natural response when food is withheld and means that calories are burned up (or used) at a slower rate. This is why some people actually put on weight while dieting.

Being healthy and feeling vital is our natural state. Don't you think it's interesting that we do not notice that we are well, we only notice when we feel unwell or uncomfortable.

Poor sleep patterns disrupt your metabolism

Let's take this a little further. Your metabolic clock signals at 8 pm that it's tired and wants you to rest and prepare for healing sleep. It's responding to sunset and the relaxing hormone, melatonin, which is triggered around this time of day. You override this signal and decide to do your housework or complete some work tasks or spend hours using the computer. Time passes, and it's now after 10 pm, and you are feeling so inspired that you don't feel like sleeping and stay up even later. When you do go to sleep, it's not restful. You toss and turn and wonder why you can't get to sleep. When you wake up you feel sluggish because you have missed out on deep healing sleep. All you want to do first thing in the morning is sleep in.

Another reason people may feel sluggish when they wake up is because they eat late at night and go to sleep with a stomach full of food. This energy for healing then has to be transferred to the digestive system for digestion rather than for rejuvenation. So, once again, your body has to make adjustments. Because you feel sluggish in the morning you skip breakfast and your metabolic clock slows down again. If you continually override the natural messages of your metabolic clock you will suffer from diminished vitality.

The importance of sleep on your metabolic clock

If you alter your sleep schedules because of lifestyle choices or work commitments, you may be endangering your health. Health studies show that if you are sleep deficient you may be putting your body on high alert. This increases the production of stress hormones and drives your blood pressure right up. You may also have elevated levels of substances in your blood that indicate inflammation, which puts you at risk of stroke, cancer or diabetes.

Eve Van Cauter of Chicago University conducted sleep research in relation to hormonal rhythms and found that a lack of sleep disrupts every physiological function in the body. Worse, 'we have nothing in our biology that allows us to adapt to this behavior.'

In a separate sleep study at the University of Chicago it was found that a lack of good sleep also disrupts the hormones ghrelin and leptin that regulate appetite. Ghrelin tells you that you are hungry and leptin tells you that you are full. Research has found that people who fail to sleep properly over-stimulate their ghrelin production, which increases their desire for food. Lack of sleep also reduces the production of leptin, which is the body's appetite suppressant. If you don't get enough sleep these two hormones get out of balance and you think you are hungry when in fact you don't need food. Further, when sleep deprived, your brain searches for carbohydrates: the University of Chicago study showed that sleep deprived people ate more sweet and starchy foods rather than protein and vegetables resulting in weight gain.

Getting sleep at the right times means not going to bed excessively late and only occasionally sleeping in. It also means having routine times for sleeping rather than getting a lot of sleep on one day and not enough the next. Getting enough sleep at the right time will assist you to have the ghrelin–leptin balance that your body needs to naturally lose weight.

A simple strategy to balance your sleep patterns is to be outside at sunrise and sunset for seven days. Set your alarm clock to wake you just before sunrise and sit outside so that the light of sunrise can trigger serotonin to be produced. Then sit outside at the end of the day when the sun sets so that your body gets a direct cue to produce melatonin to set you up for a deep, relaxing sleep.

Note for shift workers

Shift workers may not be able to follow some of *The Metabolic Clock* routines. My brother was a shift worker and I remember the difficulties he experienced trying to sleep during the day. He painted his bedroom window with thick black paint in an attempt to trick his body into believing that the sun had set. You may need to try different routines depending on your shifts to see what works best for you. One suggestion is to have your sleep time before you go to work, no matter what time of day this is. Sleep, wake up and eat and then go to work.

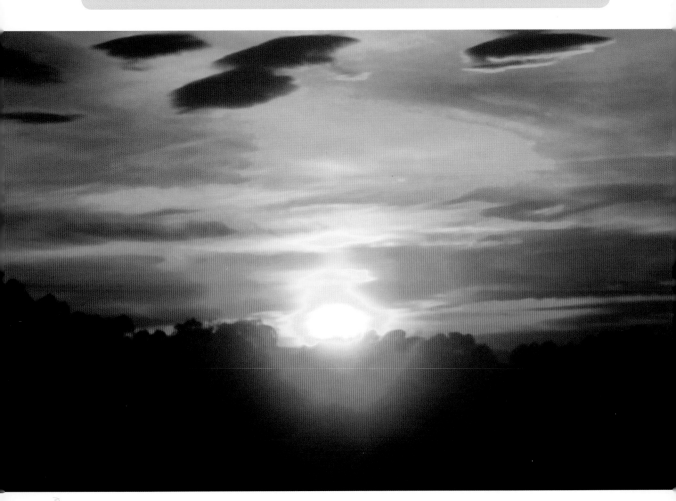

Chapter 2

Balancing your metabolic clock

When I started on my wellness journey I began to address the many unhealthy practices that had become my energy zappers. The most challenging for me was my irregular sleep and eating patterns. I took for granted the simple act of sleeping and eating at regular times. Not being mindful of these I became overtired and grumpy, lacking energy and inner peace.

At this stage in my life I was a night owl, choosing to go to bed well after midnight. I would regularly sleep restlessly and have difficulty getting up in the morning. I always woke feeling sluggish and would then have a strong coffee to get me going. It would take me a while to really get moving and I always felt behind in my day. By the end of the day I would complain that I had not had any time for myself. Almost every night I drank wine. I would then stay up late feeling unsatisfied with my personal output for the day, go to bed after midnight and wake feeling sluggish again. My natural body clock was so out of balance that I did not have enough energy at the right times: I would often feel really energized in the middle of the night and dreadfully tired in the morning.

This cycle continued for many years. My energy levels and morale were diminishing and my metabolism began to feel sluggish. After much soul-searching I realized that my lack of inner peace and unhealthy behavior was blocking me from tapping into my own natural vitality. So I decided to live my dream and make a significant change to my lifestyle – I stopped being a corporate superwoman and made a 'tree change'. I moved to the mountains with my family and pursued my dream of creating a day spa retreat and a lifestyle that created wellness.

- **Are you juggling too many agendas and trying to keep everyone happy. Do you often feel that you come last?**

- **Do you want to be fit and healthy, but feel that it's all too hard or you just simply couldn't fit another activity into your busy day?**

- **Are you constantly fighting with yourself? Do you tell yourself that you should be doing more, and then judge yourself because you aren't?**

- **Are you sabotaging your potential by overeating or some other addictive behavior?**

- **Are you finding it difficult to get to sleep at night because of the nagging negative thoughts that run through your head when you want to be sleeping?**

If you answer yes to any of these questions, your metabolic clock is in need of some balancing.

Getting in tune with your personal metabolic clock

Moving away from my hectic lifestyle and tuning into the natural rhythms of the mountains around me I quickly realized that all of God's creatures have a daily routine. They are not busy all the time. They have times to feed, times to rest and times to play. I started to think about how I could apply this natural flow to my life and realized that, unlike the animals that I was observing, I had a very random routine and with this came erratic energy levels.

Creating a balanced daily routine

How do you currently use your time and energy at any point during the day? Do you feel that you go flat-out all day? Research has shown that a highly trained athlete, let's say of Olympic standard, can only run flat out for approximately 70 metres. If you were to speak to the coach of a 200-metre or 400-metre athlete they would tell you that there is a race plan for these short distances. There has to be allowance for cruise sections of the race otherwise the athlete would 'blow up' (a term used by competitors when the very toxic lactic acid levels prevent them from continuing the run).

   If a highly trained athlete can't run flat-out for long periods of time, how can you expect to work flat-out all day and be at peak efficiency without your very own race plan, or, as I like to call it, an energy management plan? By creating your own energy management plan you will be able to balance your daily routine for maximum results to your health and wellbeing.

Balance is just as important in you as it is in nature

When your metabolic clock is out of balance you may experience unhealthy emotions, which will affect how you treat yourself and others. You may also feel that you are constantly swimming upstream and quite literally feel that you are using up a lot of energy and not really getting very far. Go with the flow of nature and the balancing act will become a lot easier to manage.

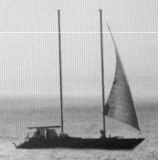

Go with the flow of nature and the balancing act will become a lot easier to manage.

Identify your energy pattern

In order to balance your body clock, you will need to identify your energy pattern from the examples below.

1. Do you regularly skip breakfast and drink lots of tea and coffee to keep you going? Are you always putting yourself last? Do you constantly deplete your energy without nurturing and nourishing your body? With a lack of nourishment and a feeling that you have to take it all on yourself, you may soon burn out and feel depleted, resentful and discouraged. Your energy pattern may look like this as you find your energy dropping throughout the day.

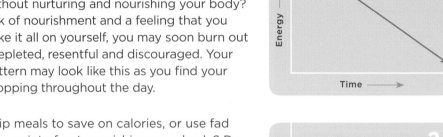

2. Do you skip meals to save on calories, or use fad diets to the point of not nourishing your body? Do you experience negative self-talk and have sugar binges? Do these all or nothing strategies and sugar binges weaken your immune system and leave you feeling moody and restless? Your energy pattern may look like this with your energy being very up and down throughout the day.

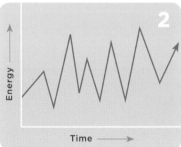

3. Are you focused, motivated and driven, but miss the early warning signs to slow down and nurture yourself? Are you so busy being driven that you have forgotten to allocate time to take care of your health? If you don't allocate time to be healthy, then you may need a lot more time to recover from being sick. Your energy pattern may look like this where you can be feeling good and then suddenly feel seriously ill.

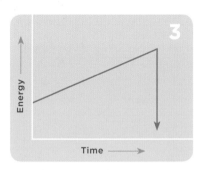

4. Do you feel overwhelmed easily and have no systems or strategies to cope or easily make changes? Do you have clutter around you and choose to hang on to things rather than deal with them? Does this overwhelm you, causing you to complain or blame others? Do you feel that the only way to feel good is to comfort eat which then leads to being overweight and overwhelming your body? Do you loop between procrastination and guilt? Your energy pattern may look like this, where you always feel sluggish and tired.

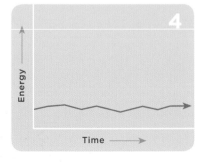

The Metabolic Clock has strategies to create effective energy patterns that will balance all the activities in your day, helping you to become fulfilled and happy. The powerful energy management and planning strategies in The Metabolic Clock are easy to follow. You will experience the right energy at the right time and feel balanced.

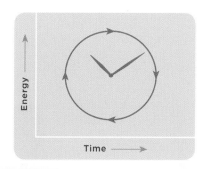

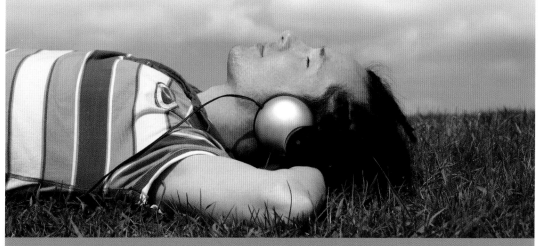

Creating more 'me time'

One of the most common desires that people have is that they would like more 'me time'. It seems really common for people to work hard all day hoping for some time to themselves at the end of the day. However, when they do get to the end of the day they are burned out, feel overwhelmed and due to a lack of energy, simply give up on the notion that they could do something for their own happiness. They dive for the sofa and begin comfort eating. It seems as though the most important person is placed last. This ineffective strategy leads to thoughts of 'what about me?' followed by feelings of resentment and unhealthy choices.

What if this pattern was switched around? What if you paid attention to yourself at the start of the day instead of at the end? What if you honoured your interests first? It's likely that you would begin your day in a much happier way and this would energise you for the day's activities. You would get to the end of the day in a much happier state because you would no longer be waiting for time for you. You will probably be keen to nourish yourself, share time with family and friends and get to bed early so that you awaken fresh and ready for more time for yourself.

Six natural cycles that are key to your metabolic clock

Balance your metabolic clock with the six natural cycles that manage appetite, energy, mood and sleep.

ENERGY CYCLE 1
6 AM–10 AM
Slow and gaining momentum

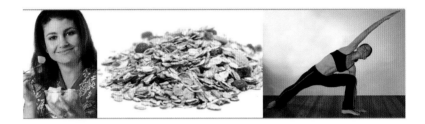

Let's begin with the sunrise cycle. From approximately 6 am to 10 am, this energy cycle is responsible for waking you gently and slowly getting you up and going.

Sunrise is your body's cue to create serotonin and other awakening hormones. If you choose to sleep in, you miss the natural energy created by these hormones. Have you ever woken up at dawn feeling alert, and then fallen asleep again for a few hours? When you wake up for the second time you feel sluggish despite having extra sleep. If you get up well after sunrise you may feel very sluggish because you are missing the use of the natural energy that is available at sunrise.

You have been fasting throughout the night. It's now time to 'break the fast' and have something to eat: which is what we know as breakfast. If you were to imagine your digestive system as a steam engine that has been resting in its bunker overnight, then the ash and burned down coals need to be emptied out of the furnace the following morning. Once cleaned out, the furnace is ready to be refuelled.

Cleansing drinks will help clear out the toxins from your overnight fast and rehydrate your digestive system. Ideal drinks are water at room temperature, freshly juiced fruit and vegetables and fresh or powdered barley or wheat grass juice. Hot water with freshly squeezed lemon juice is particularly ideal because the citric acid in lemon quickly changes an acid condition into an alkaline one, which is more ideal for helping you to feel well.

Your body now needs fuel to get it moving. Protein and low GI carbohydrates eaten at breakfast will give you a steady release of energy for the day's activities. It's really important to eat breakfast shortly after rising so that your metabolism gets activated – in other words, fuel the digestive furnace.

If you don't eat breakfast, you will still be fasting and your metabolism will slow down, leaving you feeling sluggish. If you skip breakfast and find that you have a headache coming on mid-morning, this may be because you have not broken the fast and the subsequent toxins are trying to find a way out of your system. If possible, sit in the early morning sun without sunscreen to eat your breakfast. Morning sun delivers serotonin, which is a happy hormone, and also vitamin D. A lack of vitamin D can leave you feeling tired and depressed.

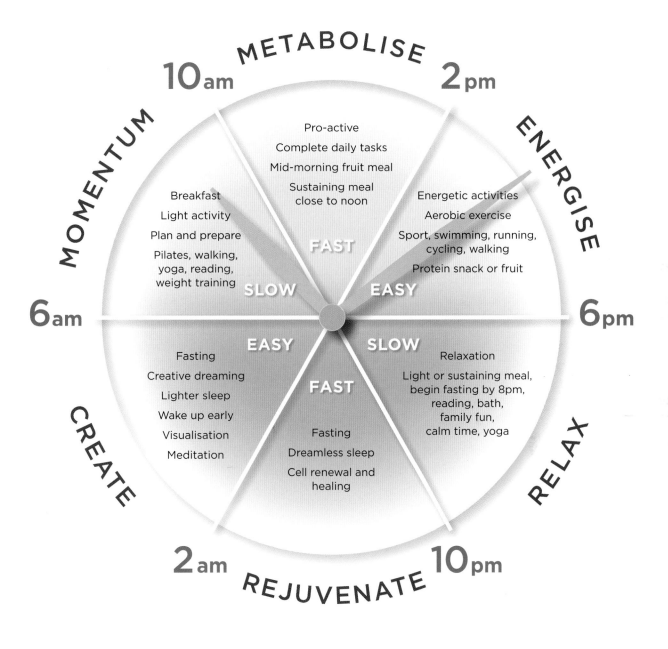

METABOLISE

10am **2pm**

MOMENTUM **ENERGISE**

6am **6pm**

Pro-active
Complete daily tasks
Mid-morning fruit meal
Sustaining meal
close to noon

Breakfast
Light activity
Plan and prepare
Pilates, walking,
yoga, reading,
weight training

FAST

Energetic activities
Aerobic exercise
Sport, swimming, running,
cycling, walking
Protein snack or fruit

SLOW **EASY**

EASY **SLOW**

Fasting
Creative dreaming
Lighter sleep
Wake up early
Visualisation
Meditation

FAST

Relaxation
Light or sustaining meal,
begin fasting by 8pm,
reading, bath,
family fun,
calm time, yoga

Fasting
Dreamless sleep
Cell renewal and
healing

CREATE **RELAX**

2am **10pm**

REJUVENATE

Many people like to rise early and exercise. If you exercise early in the morning, it's important to allow time to eat after you're done. Although you have increased your metabolic rate by exercising, by not eating a message is sent to your brain that no food is available and your body responds by slowing down the metabolism to conserve fuel. This negates your effort to speed it up.

Other morning activities can include reading, meditation, yoga, Pilates, weight training, planning or preparing and breakfast meetings. It's also important to give some thought and time into planning your evening meal. It's empowering to be coming home after a busy day knowing that your evening meal is planned.

ENERGY CYCLE 2
10 AM–2 PM
Fast and metabolizing

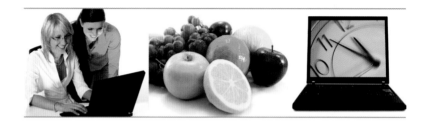

The next energy cycle is responsible for metabolizing food, distributing energy and increasing the efficiency of body processes. As the sun continues to rise and gain momentum, so too does your metabolism. The energy in this time frame more than any other encourages your metabolism to speed up, so eating food in this cycle is perfect.

The Metabolic Clock starts speeding up around 10 am, so a fruit meal at this time will process very quickly. Fruit processes in your digestive system faster than any other food, so eating fruit mid-morning is really going to speed up your metabolism. Also, raw fruit is full of life-giving enzymes that feed the healthy bacteria in your digestive tract leading to the efficient processing of food. I have often heard from people that about 20 minutes after eating fruit mid-morning they are really hungry. This is a good sign that their metabolism is working efficiently and is ready for an early lunch.

Eat two pieces of fruit at around 10 am. It is very easy and makes a great portable snack. (Pineapple contains an enzyme called bromelain, which burns fat, so this is a particularly good fruit to eat at this time to burn body fat.)

In alignment with the sun being at its hottest, eat a nourishing meal close to midday when your metabolism is still very active. This will give you the fuel for an energetic afternoon. It makes sense to have most of your daily intake of food at this time to ensure fast metabolising and also to give you energy for the rest of the day. Eat carbohydrates, protein, salads and vegetables at this time of the day (see Midday Meal ideas on p118).

If you skip lunch on a fast metabolising cycle you will be left feeling very low in energy after 2 pm when this cycle changes to being light and energetic. Your digestive furnace will lose momentum and not generate much energy.

ENERGY CYCLE 3
2 PM–6 PM
Easy, light and energetic

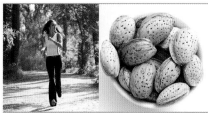
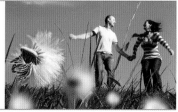

This light, energetic energy cycle is responsible for enthusiasm and movement. It is good to have a protein snack mid-afternoon. Protein satisfies the body and stops you from feeling hungry. A handful of almonds or yoghurt is a good choice. This is not a good time of the day to add carbohydrates as your need for fuel is lessening and the rationale is to use up all the carbohydrates before you go to sleep.

This is a great time of day to exercise or work on a creative project. If you are lacking the motivation to exercise in the morning, try exercising late in the afternoon because you will be feeling lighter than in the morning. It's also a good way to use up all the excess fuel created by eating carbohydrates throughout the day. Carbohydrates provide fuel only, and if you do not use all the fuel created by the digestion of carbohydrates then your body stores this as fat when you go to sleep. Aerobic exercise for 30 to 40 minutes speeds up your metabolic rate, which means that you will burn fuel faster. If you have an early dinner with very few carbohydrates you will begin to burn your body fat as fuel. Go for a run, swim, ride a bike, play sport or walk briskly at this time of the day.

It's really simple to go for a walk straight after work. Change into comfortable clothes and get out that front door. Take your partner or a friend with you. Not only will you be moving your body, you will be releasing stress from the day's activities.

ENERGY CYCLE 4
6 PM–10 PM
Slow and relaxing

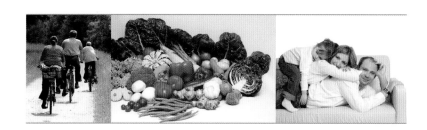

This is the beginning of nature's sunset cycle and it's a slow, relaxing cycle that is responsible for slowing you down and preparing you for much needed rest and sleep. With this comes the slowing down of your metabolism. This is why it's not recommended that you eat a large meal at this time. Many people eat a large meal laden with carbohydrates late at night only to find that they feel uncomfortable while sleeping and wake up feeling sluggish. Feeling sluggish in the morning they decide not to eat breakfast. Then a slow metabolizing pattern begins. Change the pattern, tune into the energy cycle and become more alert and energetic during the day.

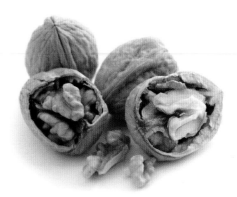

Add some walnuts to your evening meal because they are naturally high in melatonin and will help you to relax into a good night's sleep.

By not eating carbohydrates at night, you will burn body fat while you sleep.

The role of carbohydrates is to provide energy. If you eat carbohydrates at night your body will store this energy as fat while you sleep as not much energy is needed at this time. If you go to bed without eating carbohydrates then the reverse will happen and your body will burn fat for energy while you sleep. Simply put, bread, pasta, rice and noodles are best eaten at midday.

In the early evening eat a nourishing meal made up of protein and vegetables, which will provide the nutrients for building and repairing your cells. I call this a protein and enzyme-rich meal. A large raw salad provides a workout for your digestive system, which helps to speed up your metabolism. Raw salad vegetables are very low in calories so you can eat plenty of them. When you eat a big salad there is a large volume of fibre to work its way through your digestive system. In other words, this is 'the exercise program that doesn't raise a sweat'.

Raw vegetables are laden with life-giving enzymes, which act like spark plugs to fire up the many healing processes within your body. They also provide water, which helps to balance the moisture content in your colon. This is all good news for the proper functioning of your digestive system. There are also minerals and vitamins in vegetables that nourish your body and antioxidants that clean up unwanted toxins.

The good bacteria in your digestive system require feeding. Raw vegetables, especially leafy greens, ferment well creating the environment for the good bacteria to thrive. You can add a lot of variety to your meals by adding a large raw salad every day. All that chewing in your mouth gets the digestive enzymes and other chemicals activated in your digestive system, which speeds it up. Eating lighter food at night will ensure digestion is easy and you are comfortable while you are sleeping. This also means that there will be energy available for the building and repairing of cells.

If your digestive system is very sluggish you can have a fibre supplement 15 minutes before your evening meal. You will experience a feeling of fullness, which can also help you to eat a lighter meal in the evening. The fibre will also work really well during your night sleep because your digestive system will be relaxed as you sleep, which will further speed up your metabolism.

Get some 'before midnight' sleep

Getting some sleep before midnight helps your body to heal and burn body fat. This also assists in creating balance in the two hormones, ghrelin and leptin, which regulate appetite.

You may have noticed that as evening approaches you slow down and begin to unwind. Your body naturally responds to this cycle (which is aligned with the sun setting) and gets ready for sleep by producing melatonin, the relaxing hormone. However, if you do any stimulating activities in this time frame you will miss the cue that is preparing you for a relaxing sleep. You may have felt tired at 8 pm but continued doing a stimulating activity. You go to bed after 12 am feeling wide awake and at 1.30 am you still can't fall asleep. You may eventually get some sleep, however it will be a lighter sleep filled with very active and creative dreams. You will find that you wake up feeling sluggish or get up late in the morning.

It's ideal to be asleep before 10 pm while you are in the slow, relaxing energy cycle, as these are ideal circumstances for sliding into deep, dreamless sleep. I call this the sleep slide, and if you miss the sleep slide you may miss the accompanying deep sleep that is very rejuvenating. If you feel tired at 9 pm, it does not mean that you are lacking in vitality. It's natural to feel tired just before sleeping. It's also natural and possible to feel energized and awake at sunrise when the get-up-and-go hormone serotonin is produced in partnership with sunrise.

If you constantly go to bed late and deprive yourself of deep sleep, you raise the levels of the stress hormone cortisol that lifts blood sugar levels. This zaps your energy, leaving you feeling sluggish, and slows the metabolism. This unhealthy sleep cycle can reduce the production of the hormone leptin, which suppresses appetite. It can also over produce the hormone ghrelin, which tells you that you are hungry. So, even though your body may not need the fuel, you think it does, so you overeat and stay up late snacking.

ENERGY CYCLE 5
10 PM–2 AM
**Fast and
rejuvenating**

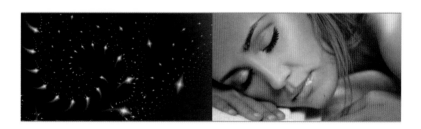

In this energy cycle, during deep sleep, you enter a fast and rejuvenating cycle, which is for cell renewal and the deep cleansing of body processes. Essentially you will be fasting throughout this cycle. It's really important to have begun your fast before you enter this cycle and this is why it's suggested that you have an early dinner and then stop eating until the morning. If you relaxed in the previous energy cycle it will be easy to enter into a deep and restful sleep.

Dreamless sleep is required for the peace of the soul

Can you remember a time when you were a child and you closed your eyes to go to sleep and slept so deeply that when you opened your eyes it seemed like you had just closed them? Dreamless sleep rejuvenates the soul and a rejuvenated soul energizes you.

Many people think that deep sleep is only required to rest and heal the body. Maybe dreamless sleep is about giving the soul a break. Think of it this way: your soul out of the body is free. Your soul in the body experiences the pressure cooker of negative thoughts and physical toxins. Maybe dreamless sleep allows the soul to be free and maybe it goes back to where it came from to be rejuvenated? Did you know that in this deep sleep cycle all of our senses are turned off? We cannot see, hear, feel or smell when the soul leaves. We all know that when we do not get deep, restful sleep our emotions change and we become moody and easily irritated. It is as though we are not at peace. The next time you feel like this during the day, plan for a good night's sleep.

SOME TIPS TO HELP YOU SLEEP DEEPLY.
- Eat a light meal early in the evening.
- Minimise carbohydrates at dinner time.
- Do not drink tea or coffee after 4 pm.
- Do not activate your mind by working after 8 pm.
- Engage in any activity that is relaxing for you.
- If anything is on your mind, write it down in a notebook before you go to bed, and decide not to think about it until the morning.
- Play calming music before going to bed.
- Have a shower or a bath before going to bed.
- Sit in a dark room and relax before going to bed.
- Be in bed close to or before 10 pm.

ENERGY CYCLE 6
2 AM–6 AM
Easy, light and creative

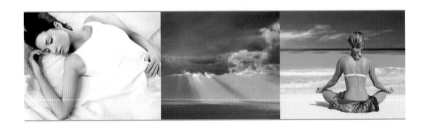

This cycle is responsible for bringing you out of deep sleep and gently waking you. Your mind begins to become activated from its dreamless state with creative dreaming. When you wake up at sunrise, get up and override the thoughts that want to keep you in the dreamy state. Sunrise or dawn is a perfect time of day to have quality time with yourself or with your partner. If you are not finding it easy to get up early, then go to bed earlier.

Meditation is an excellent pre-dawn activity that helps you towards peace of mind. Studies have shown that people who meditate regularly cope better with the stress in their lives. Many people choose to get up before this creative cycle ends and engage in creative projects, like writing or study. This is also a great time of day to visualise or daydream. Use your imagination to think creatively about your goals. Think about all the things you are grateful for. This will certainly put a smile on your face and you will begin your day in a happy way.

People who like exercising in the morning like to start before this easy and light cycle ends. I have met many people who get up at 5 am to go running or work out in the gym as they enjoy exercising and feeling the lightness of this energy cycle.

Putting it all together to reset your body clock

Use the natural energy cycles of The Metabolic Clock and create a daily routine that brings more balance and energy to your day. The Metabolic Clock is a 24-hour clock. Each time frame affects the next. All six time frames will come into balance if you focus on the activities in each section.

1. Wake up at sunrise and gently stretch your body. Sit quietly for 3 minutes and visualize what you would like to experience in your life. Meditate and think of what you are grateful for.
2. Start the day with a cleansing drink. This will rehydrate your body and help to cleanse the toxins from your overnight fast. Ideal cleansing drinks are water at room temperature, boiled water with freshly squeezed lemon juice, fresh or powdered barley or wheat grass juice and raw, freshly juiced fruits or vegetables.
3. Exercise if you like to exercise in the morning. This is a good time of the day for yoga and Pilates exercises, which encourage the natural flow of energy in the body.
4. Eat breakfast so that your metabolism gets moving. Sit in the early morning sun while you eat your breakfast. Morning sun helps your body to create serotonin, which is known as the happy hormone.
5. Eat fruit mid-morning to speed up your metabolism and fill your body with life-giving enzymes.
6. Eat a nourishing meal close to midday when your metabolism is very active. This will give you the fuel for an energetic afternoon and keep your metabolism moving.
7. If hungry, have a mid-afternoon protein snack.
8. Do energetic exercise or walk to burn off excess fuel from carbohydrates late in the afternoon.
9. Eat a light meal of protein and vegetables in the early evening. Then begin your fast and do not eat again until morning. Eat your meal slowly and enjoy relaxed conversation with the people around you.
10. Allow yourself to relax and prepare for a restful night's sleep. Do not drink tea or coffee or engage in activities that stimulate the mind. Ensure that you are in bed well before midnight to ensure you experience deep sleep that rejuvenates and heals.

It's important to remember that your body functions naturally when in tune with this 24-hour clock. Any practices that you may have that do not match this clock are simply chosen behaviours that can be altered. Allow a couple of weeks for adjustment of the energy cycles and enjoy feeling lighter and more energised. You will find that you naturally wake up at sunrise, power through your day, sleep deeply and have more time and energy for the things you love.

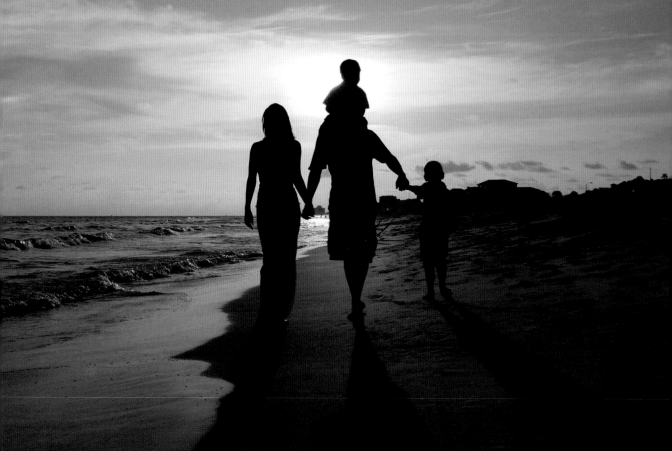

Have more time and energy
for the things you love.

Chapter 3

Revitalise your digestive system

In all my years of mentoring people on their health, what stands out most is the relationship between vitality and the proper functioning of the digestive system. I have seen many people shed body fat quickly and easily when they have brought their unhealthy digestive system back into balance.

There are three things that dramatically affect the efficiency of your digestive system.
1. Being stressed slows down the metabolism.
2. A clogged colon disrupts the absorption of nutrients and weakens the immune system.
3. An imbalance of digestive bacteria disrupts digestion and can create food cravings.

There are six daily practices that will bring your digestive system back into balance.
1. Eat slowly and thoroughly chew food before swallowing.
2. Relax as you eat.
3. Eat fibre-rich food.
4. Eat enzyme-rich food.
5. Boost good bacteria.
6. Drink water and eat water-rich plant foods.

1 Eat slowly and thoroughly chew food before swallowing

The digestive tract can be described from mouth to anus as a 25-foot hose. Its function is to turn what we eat into microscopic particles that the cells use for energy to perform their many functions and then to eliminate what isn't required.

Thoroughly chewing food allows for the system of digestion to begin by breaking down the food into smaller pieces. The receptors in your mouth send messages to the brain, which then organizes for the stomach to get the chemicals ready to begin to break down the food in the next stage. If you are too busy to chew your food thoroughly then you are missing out on the first part of the digestive process. This makes it more difficult for the stomach to break down the food and can be overwhelming for it. When anything is overwhelmed, it slows down.

This is why it is important to eat your food very slowly and chew thoroughly before swallowing. Try putting your knife and fork down between mouthfuls to remind you to eat slowly.

Louise had suffered from reflux for five years. Although not life threatening, she always felt uncomfortable after eating. She had been tested thoroughly with every associated medical test and the results were inconclusive. No one could identify the problem or solution. During a mentoring session Louise realized that she always gulped down her food really fast without chewing and often ate on the run. After a few weeks of making simple adjustments to thoroughly chew her food and always sit down to eat, her reflux magically disappeared.

Give your attention to what you are eating and how you are eating.
If you eat while you are working at your desk, you may find that
you eat more food than you realize. This is simply because you
have not noticed how much you are eating.

2 Relax as you eat

The digestive tract operates like a muscle, contracting and releasing, passing the food through. When you are stressed, the muscles of the colon react by squeezing the colon into an unnatural shape and the process stops or stalls and so does the processing of the food eaten. What this means is that you slow down your metabolism.

The next time you feel stressed, pause for a moment and notice if you feel tense in your gut. The digestive system has as many nerve endings as the spine, so it makes sense that if you are feeling stressed, anxious or nervous, the nerve endings in your gut respond to this stress. This can easily produce bouts of constipation.

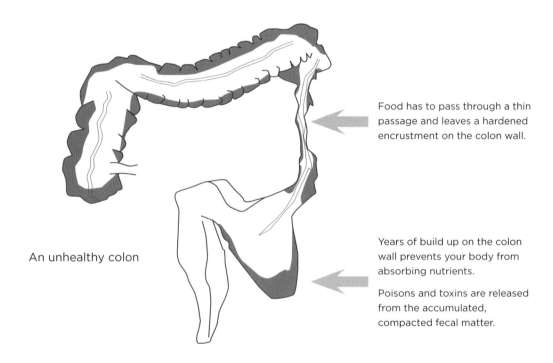

An unhealthy colon

Food has to pass through a thin passage and leaves a hardened encrustment on the colon wall.

Years of build up on the colon wall prevents your body from absorbing nutrients.

Poisons and toxins are released from the accumulated, compacted fecal matter.

SLOW DOWN TO SPEED UP YOUR DIGESTIVE SYSTEM
This is the case when you want to speed up your digestive system. When you slow down and relax, your digestive system speeds up in response, releasing any blockages in your colon. This is why eating in a relaxed and calm environment is good for digestion.

Dealing with stress by allowing time for relaxation, especially when you are eating, is going to assist in keeping your metabolism moving.

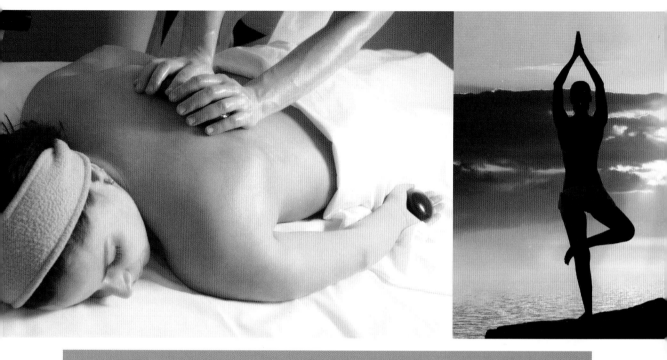

Some helpful relaxation strategies to alleviate stress

- Relax in a bath.
- Make meal times relaxing and always sit down to eat.
- Treat yourself to a relaxing massage regularly.
- Spend creative time on your favorite non-work activities.
- Walk along the beach.
- Do some gardening.
- Play a musical instrument.
- Join a meditation or yoga class.
- Sit in the early morning sun.
- Watch a funny movie.
- Get up before everybody else and sit quietly, focusing your attention within.
- Explore something new for the day and get away from your usual surroundings.
- Schedule some fun times with family and friends.
- Go to bed early to allow for dreamless sleep.
- Make time for moments of stillness.
- Listen to your breathing and feel the life energy inside your body.
- Eat green plant food. Green is the most relaxing color to the human eye.
- Take a silent walk in a lush, green forest.
- Give appreciation and kindness to yourself and everyone you meet.
- Many times a day, focus on your gut. Are you holding tension here? If you are, take a deep breath and say to yourself several times, 'relax, release and let it go'.

3 Eat fibre-rich food

Everything that you put into your body has to be digested. Eating food that is as close to its natural state as possible, rather than processed food, helps to keep your digestive system functioning properly.

Maximum assimilation of nutrients in the small intestine can only happen if the intestinal walls are free of waste buildup.

The lining of the digestive tract is covered in millions of villi or minute finger-like structures that have a blood supply. It is through these villi that nutrients are absorbed into your bloodstream and carried to nourish the rest of your body. If you were to unravel the entire surface area of your digestive tract it would almost cover a tennis court, and if you imagine the villi as grass, then you would have a grass tennis court.

This grass tennis court needs watering and feeding to thrive. Imagine watering the grass tennis court with cola, coffee, alcohol, tea and mostly feeding it with processed food and sugary snacks. These foods contain no nourishment or fibre. Without fibre these foods can sit for a long period of time waiting to be processed. The result of this can be a buildup of a tar-like coating on the intestinal walls. Your grass tennis court will look more like a bitumen tennis court and when this happens, absorption of nutrients will not be easy through the sticky tar on the surface.

The impacted matter then begins to block the colon or even twist it, making it difficult for food to pass through and for nutrients to be absorbed. This impacted matter can putrefy and release toxins and poisons. This toxicity and subsequent lack of vitality can be the beginning of weight gain and chronic illness if not corrected.

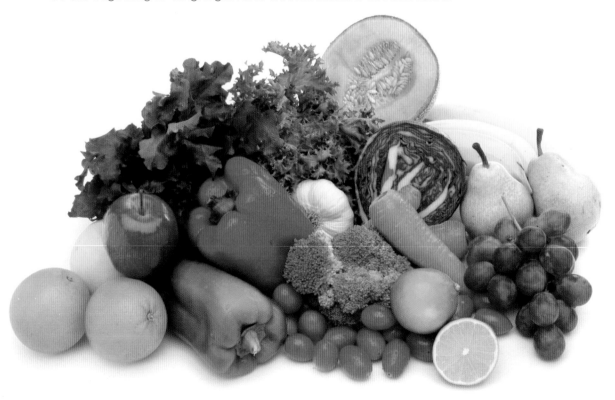

Seventy per cent of the body's immune system is found in the digestive tract

The lymphatic system is your body's defence system (see more information on the lymphatic system in Chapter 4 'Move your body to feel good about yourself'). Its role is to engulf foreign bodies, bacteria, viruses and debris and safely transport them out of your body. The lymphatic system runs parallel to the arteries and veins in the body and the lymph fluid contained in the system is a colorless fluid that transports white blood cells, which fight foreign invaders and infection.

Now, imagine that 70 per cent of the lymphatic system is in your digestive tract running parallel to the millions of villi that absorb the nourishment from your food. If you have impacted matter on the lining of your colon you are not only blocking the absorption of nourishment, you are also blocking the lymphatic system from its defence duties.

You do not have to be a scientist to realize that this is going to affect your health, as you may not be able to fight off infections as easily if you have a clogged colon. The good news is that the colon is quick to heal as long as it is given the correct raw materials to work with.

Fibre has long been recognized as one of the best elements for maintaining regularity of the bowel and keeping intestinal walls free of waste build-up. Eating fibre-rich foods reduces the transit time of food through the bowel, resulting in a more efficient and thorough evacuation of waste materials. Raw, fibre-rich foods provide a workout for the digestive system, getting things moving and speeding up the metabolism. Fibre-rich foods are generally plant foods: fruits and vegetables, nuts and seeds, wholegrains and legumes.

Adding a little extra fibre to your diet

If your digestive system needs a kick-start, add one heaped teaspoon of a fibre supplement taken in water 15 minutes before your evening meal. This will give you a feeling of being full. Then, eat a light dinner and during sleep your digestive system will relax, making it easy for the fibre to clean out a clogged colon. It will also reshape any stressed or squeezed parts of the colon bringing it back to its healthy, natural shape. (Note: A fibre supplement is not a replacement for eating fibre-rich foods.)

4 Eat enzyme-rich food

Enzymes are the sparks that start the chemical reactions needed for our bodies to live. An enzyme is a biocatalyst, which is the trigger to make something happen or work faster. I consider enzymes to be the body's spark plugs. This is good news because eating raw food that is full of live enzymes will spark your metabolism to move faster. It's also interesting to note that in Western cultures we are eating a lot of packaged and processed foods that have little or no enzymes. Is it any wonder we are experiencing diminished vitality?

Everything you put into your stomach requires digestive enzymes to process it. We only have a limited number of digestive enzymes when we are born, so it's important to replenish enzymes by eating raw food (as raw food is rich in enzymes). If we don't replenish the enzymes then we run the risk of the early onset of degenerative diseases and premature ageing.

You may be of an age to remember that before the age of 30, it was easy to stay out all night and trash your body. You would have felt that you recovered really well and may even have felt invincible. However, as the years progressed, you noticed that you could no longer stay out all night and still feel energized the next day. You might have put this change down to growing older.

What's really happening is that your body is being quickly depleted of the enzymes it was born with. By the time your body reaches 30, its natural intelligence reassesses the way it's dealing out the enzymes to heal the damage from your partying ways. It senses that if it keeps this up all the enzymes that you were born with will be depleted by the time you are 40. As it begins to pace the release of the enzymes, you find that you don't recover quite so quickly from a big night out.

Enzymes could be called the youth juice.
Without them, you age really quickly.

Foods full of enzymes can be thought of as live food. Enzymes from raw food speed up the metabolism and create a beneficial environment for good bacteria to grow and thrive. It's as easy as:

- eating a raw salad every day
- starting your day with a fresh juice – freshly juiced fruit or vegetables first thing in the morning will fill your digestive system with antioxidants and enzymes that will kick start your metabolism
- putting fresh herbs over your cooked food, like chopped parsley on your poached eggs
- nibbling on raw vegetables while you are preparing dinner and chewing them well – give the kids a platter of chopped raw carrot, celery, sugar snap peas and cucumber just before dinner (I find that my kids enjoy vegetables raw, rather than cooked).

5 Boost good bacteria

The secret to good health lies with the friendly bacteria found in the intestinal tract. These friendly bacteria regulate the digestive processes, reducing the levels of toxic bacteria that can cause ill health. The digestive tract is a living ecosystem with billions of micro-organisms. Like any ecosystem, it thrives when the balance is right. But if it goes out of balance, the system doesn't function as efficiently as it is designed to. This imbalance results in a lack of vitality.

The friendly bacteria keep the bad bacteria from growing out of control, providing you create the right environment in your gut for this to happen. The presence of active bacteria in the gut aids the digestive process by fermenting foods so that the nourishment of the food can be easily absorbed through the intestinal lining.

You can create a healthy environment for the good bacteria in your digestive system by eating raw vegetables, especially green leaves, fruit, nuts, seeds and wholegrains. Adding a probiotic supplement to your nutritional strategy will also encourage the healthy bacteria in your digestive tract.

Many practices of the Western diet destroys the good bacteria. This inevitably slows down the body's metabolism.

Common things that kill good bacteria in the body are:
- stress
- alcohol
- antibiotics and birth control pills
- steroids and hormone drugs
- pain-relief drugs
- coffee and tea
- preservatives and additives.

CANDIDA

Another culprit that can rob you of digestive wellness is an overgrowth of candida. Many ailments and even weight problems can be due to an overgrowth of candida in your digestive tract. Candida is a yeast-like fungus that is present in everyone's body but goes out of control when the body's balance is upset.

Candida is only intended to overgrow and get out of control when the body dies, when its characteristics change in order to break down the body. Candida out of balance and overgrown while a person is alive is very disruptive, and not what nature intended.

If you wake up in the morning with a thick white coating on your tongue then chances are this is candida. This overgrowth can affect you from your head to your toes. Other symptoms include migraines, toenail fungus, pain and inflammation in organs and joints. It can also cause problems with your mind and emotions. On the skin it can present as eczema and hives. Generally it will give you poor digestion, thrush, bloating and low energy.

Candida thrives on sugar, refined carbohydrates and the yeast in breads, pastries, pizza and alcohol, so minimise these foods and increase your intake of fresh food. You can also boost your good bacteria with a probiotic supplement, which contains the good bacteria necessary for healthy flora in your intestines. Eating a diet rich in fibre and adding a fibre supplement will help to clear the intestinal lining of candida as it dies off.

6 Drink water and eat water-rich plant foods

Once food is broken down and absorbed into your bloodstream, anything left goes into the colon. The colon's function is to absorb water and the remaining nutrients, forming

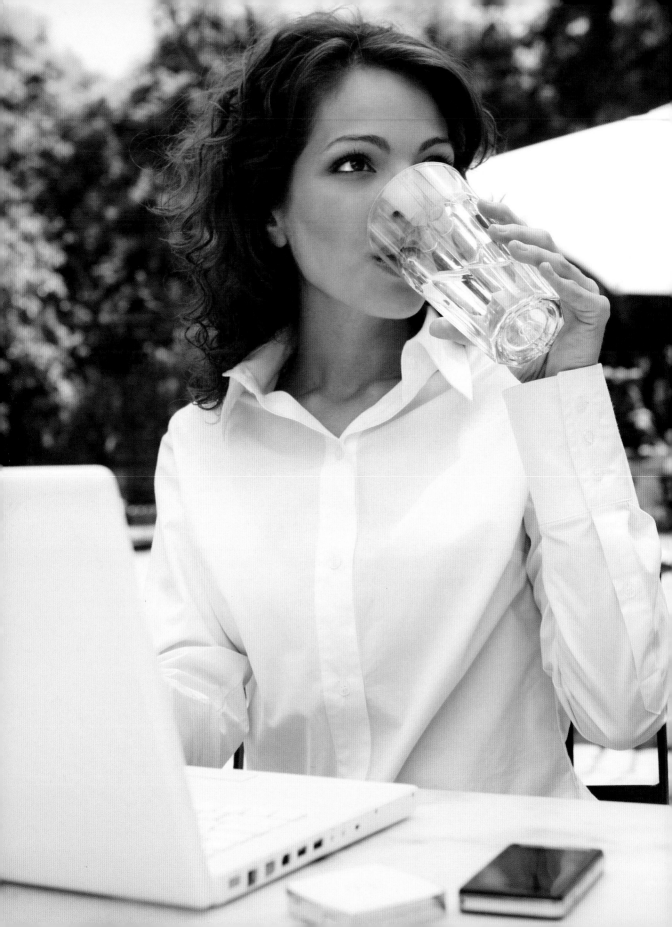

a soft stool. The further through your digestive system the food goes, the more water is absorbed. If you don't drink water and eat water-rich fruits and vegetables, you may be setting yourself up for very dry stools or even uncomfortable constipation.

Eating two pieces of fruit mid-morning and vegetable combinations twice a day will provide moisture to your colon. Drinking 6 to 8 glasses of water each day will keep your digestive system moist and comfortable. Drink water between meals rather than with your meals as water dilutes the stomach acid that is required for breaking down the hard protein coating around certain foods.

Why should I drink water?

Your body contains approximately 11 litres (23 pints) of tissue fluid. This tissue fluid surrounds the cells of the body and bathes them. It delivers communication and the raw materials that the cells require to function. It also removes metabolic waste material.

If you drink 6 to 8 glasses of water a day, you'll maintain an ideal level of tissue fluid. If you become dehydrated, how can you expect this tissue fluid to be efficient?

Imagine your level of tissue fluid dropping to 7 litres (15 pints). The level of toxins would become very intense, possibly giving you a headache. Communication to nerve cells would slow down making your reaction time and energy levels diminish. Your brain cells would be foggy, making it more difficult to think clearly or make decisions, and your digestive system would become sluggish.

Weight loss and toxins

Your body stores toxins in fat tissue. This will affect your overall health. You may have some signs of toxicity.

When you begin a healthy eating program and burn body fat, your cells begin to eliminate the toxic substances. The process your body goes through to get rid of toxins is called detoxification.

Your body always goes for quality. When the food coming in is of a high quality, the body will discard the present tissue because it wants to make room for tissue created by the higher quality food. In this way, the tissues are being cleansed and the toxins are being released into the bloodstream to be removed from the body.

Put simply, these toxins are harmful to the cells of your body and a little discomfort to eliminate them can save you years of illness and pain.

This elimination may result in headaches. Often toxins are eliminated through the skin, resulting in rashes or skin problems. You may also feel a lack of energy. This is temporary and although you may feel slightly unwell, you will soon feel fantastic as the new cells will be healthier and your body will not be carrying around as many toxins.

How long the symptoms last and how severe they are will depend on the lifestyle you had before making a positive change. While most people do not experience these symptoms, it's important to know that this is part of the healing process and the discomfort will vanish in a few days. The hardest thing for many people to do is to accept that they are not sick and to realise that their body is cleansing itself.

Supporting the detoxification process

The following simple strategies will support the detox process and get you on the path to health and vitality.

- Rest. Give your body as much energy as possible to do its cleansing.
- Eat lots of fruit and vegetables.
- Drink plenty of water.
- Have a detoxifying bath with Epsom salts or sea salt.
- Use a sauna or steam room.
- Get some fresh air in a natural environment.
- Be gentle to yourself.
- Go for a walk. Movement activates the lymphatic system to eliminate toxins.

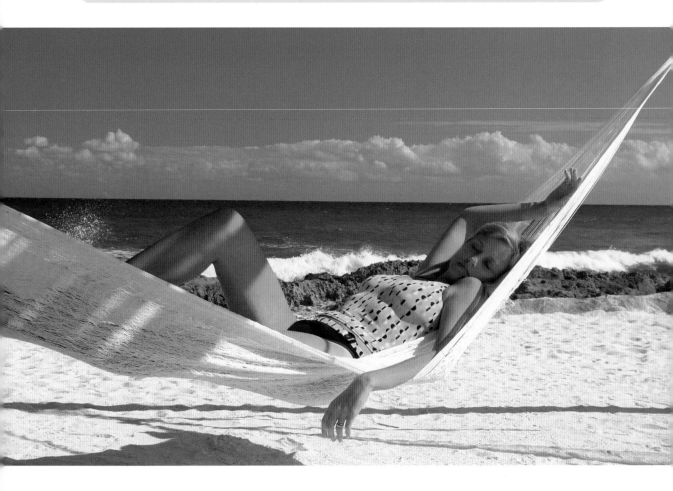

Chapter 4

Move your body and feel good about yourself

I meet many people who have no desire to exercise heavily or raise a sweat to lose weight. You can certainly lose weight with *The Metabolic Clock* without exercising, but moving your body is essential for reasons other than losing weight.

Exercising for a healthy immune system

Your body naturally knows how to release toxins and does this in many ways. One of these is via the lymphatic system (this was discussed earlier in Chapter 3 on revitalizing your digestive system). The lymph system, or immune system, has no pump or beat of its own and so needs movement to activate it and circulate the toxins. Moving your body primes the pump. It's also well proven that to help ill people recover quickly, they need to move their bodies.

> **Joseph Pilates was born in 1880. He was a sickly child and as he got older, he became determined to improve his health. He made it his life's work to find out about all forms of fitness and exercise. Not only did he regain his health, he dedicated his life to helping others, creating the Pilates system of exercise.**
>
> **What's most interesting is his work at a British hospital during World War I. Understanding the importance of keeping the body moving for a healthy immune system, he created pulley systems with ropes so that bedridden war patients could move their arms and legs. When a deadly influenza came through the hospital, the patients that had kept their lymphatic system moving did not contract this illness.**

Your digestive system is lined with lymphatic tissue, which is a series of vessels that transport waste products out of the body. There are lymph nodes in your neck, armpit and groin that are like docking stations where the lymphatic fluid deposits the waste products and toxins for removal out of the body.

How the nodes remove toxins out of the body is via valves that open and close to pass the fluid along. Since the valves do not have a pump of their own, they need the surrounding muscles to contract and release, which in turn creates the pumping action that keeps the lymphatic fluid moving. When you move your arms and legs you activate these muscles. The simple act of walking will get this process working.

Change how you feel instantly by moving your body

*If your body came with an owner's manual it would say,
'Move me and you'll feel good!'*

I remember some time ago, during a busy and stressful time, I was being grumpy with my family. My partner turned to me and said, 'For goodness sake, go for a run!'

My partner was right. Exercising was the activity that would allow me to reset my thinking. I went for a run, filled my lungs with oxygen, cleared my head of judgemental language and came home in a much happier state, something my beloved family deserved.

Moving your body or exercising is vital if you approach it first to feel good and then to look good. On this basis, why wouldn't you choose it? And it's a quick way to change your emotional state. When you move your body to feel good about yourself, this propels you to want to drink water, eat healthy food, communicate, mix with people and generally get other aspects of your life moving too.

Exercising is a great way to neutralise negative emotions and quickly create vital energy. The equation is quite simple – exercise to feel good about yourself and you might just change your body shape as an added bonus!

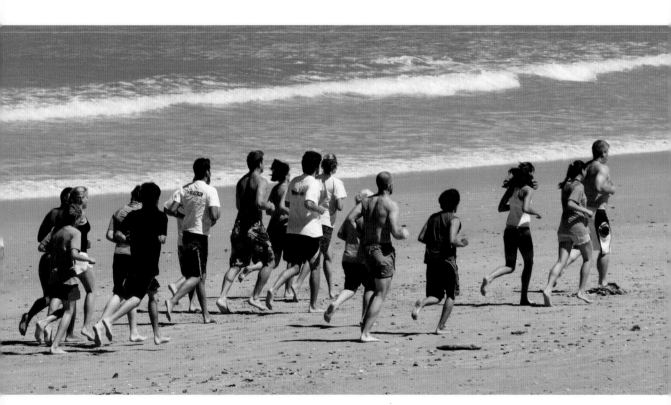

Exercise to have fun

Have you heard the saying all work and no play can make you dull? If you are feeling like this then you will possibly benefit from adopting the practice of play.

When you watch children play, they immerse themselves in the activity and use all of their physical strength to climb, crawl, run, jump, wrestle and laugh. Children literally throw themselves into whatever activity they are doing and show a strong desire to participate.

So, what has happened to you as an adult? Have you used growing up as an excuse to stop moving your body and playing? Reverse this by reintroducing small playful activities every day. This could be going on a bike ride with your kids, walking the dog, wrestling with your kids or your partner, ice-skating, shooting hoops, enjoying a hit of tennis, joining a sporting club or a swimming squad.

There are lots of ways to move your body and play. The important thing is to find what you like. It might be as simple as joining a yoga, Pilates or dance class. You might join a running squad and plan to do a fun run. There are many styles of martial arts to choose from and most fitness centres offer a variety of exercise classes. Get some friends together for regular walks.

Any of these activities will energise you and create a healthy state of mind.

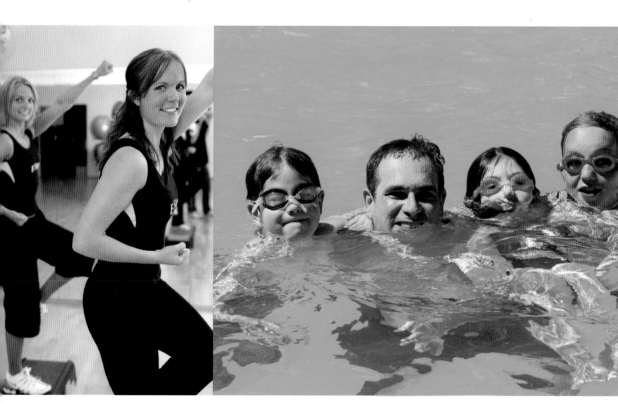

Burning body fat versus losing weight

Dieting can result in a loss of muscle as well as body fat, so doesn't always lead to a well-shaped body. On the other hand, building muscle while burning body fat is the most efficient way to re-shape your body.

When I was a young girl, I recall watching a neighbor who was a large woman. She decided that she wanted to burn body fat and did not have the financial resources to hire a personal trainer or even to join a gym. Her reasons for transforming her body must have been compelling because each night after work she skipped with a skipping rope for one hour while I watched her disciplined approach from over the fence.

Her determination paid off and her skipping eventually burned off 20 kilos of body fat. I remember feeling very inspired by her simple and effective approach to shedding body fat and the success of her transformation.

Exercise will definitely speed up your metabolism because it increases your basal metabolic rate. This is the speed that your metabolism burns fuel. Speeding this up means that you will burn fuel fast and, even better, your body will burn excess body fat for fuel.

The most efficient type of exercise for overall fitness

All types of exercise will help you to feel good about yourself. However, in my experience, there is one type of exercise that is the most efficient at speeding up your basal metabolic rate and therefore burning body fat. This is running non-stop for at least 30 minutes. It's an inexpensive and natural activity.

For many people, running for 30 minutes or more triggers endorphins, the hormones that give you a sense of wellbeing. This is known as the runner's high. Running also uses nearly every muscle in your body when you do it. It is also an aerobic activity. This means that the blood is pumped more quickly around the body, which increases the oxygen uptake to the cells. In a nutshell, running gets you and your body processes moving. Running is not essential to *The Metabolic Clock* progam, however; if you are able to run it will fast track you to your weight loss and fitness goals.

Many people who do weight-training sessions at the gym can feel unhappy with the rate that they burn off their body fat. Weight training has its place in a fitness program because it builds muscle. However, when you add three 30-minute runs per week you will achieve your fat-burning goals more quickly.

You can start by walk/running. Set out and when you feel warmed up, break into a slow jog for about 1 minute, then walk for about 4 minutes. Continue this for about 30 minutes. Each week, aim to increase the run sections until you replace the walking with the running.

When I met Fiona, her goal was to lose 40 kilos (88 pounds) of body fat. She was very sad and angry having experienced some tragedies in her life and as a result she over-ate. She was in denial about her ballooning weight until some health issues meant that she had to make some lifestyle changes.

I remember Fiona approaching me at a Metabolic Clock program. She asked for help but said that the thought of exercising was too overwhelming at that stage in her life. I made the simple suggestion of asking Fiona to get off the tram two stops before she arrived at work and walk for just a little bit each day.

A year later I bumped into her at a supermarket. She looked fantastic and had shed much of her unwanted body fat. What surprised me most was that she had enjoyed her walks to work so much that the walks had been upgraded to runs. Fiona was now able to run for 3 kilometres (2 miles) and enjoyed it so much that she was considering training for a fun run.

Using *The Metabolic Clock* strategies had increased Fiona's energy levels. She then felt like exercising, and the more she exercised the better she felt.

Good reasons to start running

- Running increases your basal metabolic rate so that you burn fuel faster.
- It fills your body with oxygen and happy hormones, making you feel good.
- You can outrun your stress.
- It clears the head of negative thoughts.
- Running improves thinking and memory function.
- It can be very social. Find some regular training partners or join a running club.
- Running improves muscle definition.
- It slows down the ageing process and promotes the body to produce human growth hormone, which strengthens bones.

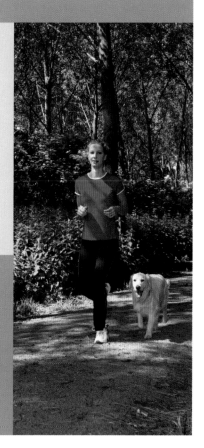

Research indicates that running can help you to live longer with less disability. A study at Stanford University School of Medicine revealed that out of 538 runners and 423 non-runners, there was less disability in the runners. They also found it easier to perform everyday tasks. Twenty years later, 85 per cent of the runners were still alive and 66 per cent of the non-runners were living. The runners had healthier bone mass and better cardiovascular health.

Fitness safety check

Before starting on any exercise program you will need to get a check-up with your doctor. This will give you an idea about your current state of health. Results from your check-up will also give you something to measure your progress against.

Book exercise times in with yourself

Doing this makes a big difference. There is always going to be some distraction that will give you reason not to exercise. To minimise these distractions, put your exercise times in your diary just as you would when making any other appointment – except this one is not negotiable.

Booking your exercise times into your weekly schedule:

- **helps you to actually commit time**
- **ensures your exercise is consistent with your goals**
- **allows you to organise your time, especially if you have people supporting you, such as personal trainers or exercise buddies.**

Every day that you exercise, record what you did and what performance indicators you used so that you can track your progress.

My favorite exercise tip is for when you really don't feel like exercising and you just can't imagine having the energy to get started. Simply commit to getting dressed to exercise and then decide if you will. What I have found is that once I am in my exercise gear I say to myself, 'I am dressed for it, I might as well do it.' Often this session is one of my better ones.

Chapter 5

Nourishment strategies for maximum energy

If you don't make time to be healthy, then at some point in your life you may need a lot of time to recover from being sick.

Being healthy is a natural state

When I was growing up it was rare to see an overweight kid. I also remember that soft drink (soda) was really only a treat at parties. We walked to school and played outside. Takeaway was a rare treat on holidays and meat and three vegetables was a common meal. There were no pre-packaged foods so we didn't have to read labels on all the food we bought. Our mothers and grandmothers handed down healthy recipes and we enjoyed family meals together. How did we go from a naturally healthy nation to a nation with more health issues and obesity than 20 years ago?

Western culture has delivered so many practices and foods that are not natural to us. As a result, obesity and a general lack of vitality occur, often due to sluggish metabolisms. Put simply, it's not another diet that is needed, it's getting back to what nature intended.

We are what we eat.

If your food intake is mainly made up of highly processed food with no nutritional value, what will your body look and feel like? If you eat fresh, natural foods, what will your health and energy levels be like? The answer to this question is fairly straightforward. So why are most Western cultures faced with enormous health issues that are diet-related? It's very simple: health is a personal choice.

As individuals we have to take responsibility for our own wellness.

Would you take a quantum leap towards feeling healthy?

There was a time when I consumed large amounts of soft drink (soda), caffeine, alcohol and foods made from white flour. When I finally found the courage to say no to these foods my health quickly improved. Doing without these foods for 3 months gave me a quantum leap towards feeling healthy. Now I only include these foods in my diet very occasionally.

The carbonation, or fizz, in soft drink (soda) disrupts your stomach acid, making it harder to digest your food. There is absolutely no nutritional value in soft drink (soda). The chemicals and colourings are toxic to your body and the high dose of sugar causes a rapid rise in blood sugar, resulting in the release of insulin from the pancreas into the bloodstream. If the pancreas is over-stimulated over a long period of time, it may become exhausted and type 2 diabetes may develop.

Did you know that it takes 33 glasses of water to balance out the acidity of one glass of soft drink (soda)? Diet soft drink (soda) is just as bad for your health. Even though they don't contain sugar, it is the artificial sweeteners that are disruptive to your health.

Caffeine in any form creates a dramatic rise in blood sugar levels. If you really enjoy your coffee, think about limiting the amount you have each day.

The health benefits of alcohol consumption are debatable. All I know is that I feel a lot healthier when I don't have it. While you are in the beginning stages of burning body fat and getting healthier, challenge yourself to have alcohol-free days each week or you might like to try seven days without alcohol and see if you feel more energised.

White flour has no nutritional value and also sends your blood sugar levels very high. Replace white flour products with wholegrain ones and you will discover a significant effect on your fat burning and digestive health.

As I've mentioned earlier in Chapter 3, eating raw food is one of the ways to nourish the body and boost your energy levels. Fresh food has a life force that provides a workout for your digestive system, speeding up your metabolism. If possible, purchase organic produce including free-range meats and eggs. They are more flavourful and are likely to contain less toxic chemicals. You don't need to go completely organic but maybe aim for 25 per cent of your diet to be organic for starters. Another option and guarantee of really fresh food is to grow your own – even if it is just herbs, salad leaves, spinach or cherry tomatoes.

Lentils are not for everyone

Only you know what it's like to be you. The way you think, what you feel, and how a particular food affects your body is an individual experience. You are the best person to create your healthy eating strategy. If you eat a certain food and have a negative reaction to that food, then your body is telling you that this particular food is not right for your body.

One of the mothers at my son's school commented that she was experiencing severe digestive problems and that there was inflammation in her bowel. She was on a waiting list to have a colon check. I had remembered from previous conversations that she was a vegetarian and that she ate mostly lentils, pasta, polenta and homemade wheat bread. I suggested that she change what she was eating for a couple of weeks. She stopped eating lentils and replaced the wheat and corn products with spelt flour products and over the next month experienced a full recovery. Her digestive system wasn't diseased, it was stressed with trying to cope with foods that it had trouble digesting.

My key food choices

The important message regarding food choices is that if something isn't working for you, change it.

With so much information about what is healthy I became overwhelmed with all the choices. Over the years I've refined some key food choices and they have become the five categories of food that I include in my diet every day because of their ability to nourish and energise.

GOOD QUALITY PROTEIN

Protein is required for the repair and growth of muscles, organs, skin, hair and nails. It's a basic building block used to rebuild cells where and when they are needed. What's interesting is that calcium is also found in many protein foods. The protein from eating oily fish also delivers essential fatty acids.

Quite simply, protein satisfies your appetite.

Protein stimulates the release of gut signals that dull your appetite. This leaves you feeling satisfied instead of hungry. Whether you decide to be a vegetarian or a meat eater, you may consider the value of eating some type of protein with every meal.

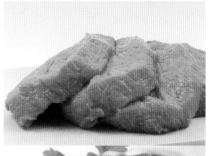

Examples of good quality protein include:

- salmon, sardines, tuna, mackerel, trout, deep-sea fish
- lean beef
- lean lamb
- free-range chicken and turkey
- rabbit
- free-range eggs
- sunflower seeds, sesame seeds, pepitas
- almonds, walnuts, pecans, Brazil nuts, macadamias
- tofu
- lentils, chickpeas, kidney beans, lima beans, cannellini beans, borlotti beans
- quinoa
- protein powder
- dairy foods in the form of natural yoghurt, goat's feta, ricotta and feta (if you are concerned about your fat intake you can choose low-fat dairy – I prefer foods that are not processed and choose dairy products in their most natural state)

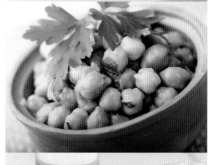

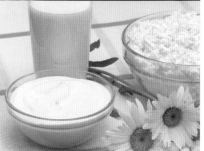

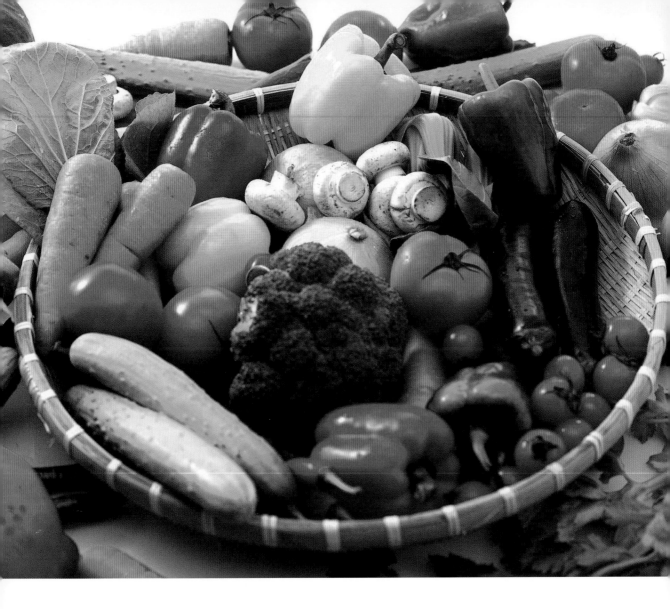

PLANT FOOD

The major part of this food category is fruits and vegetables because they are mineral- and vitamin-rich. Plant foods are nature's anti-inflammatory agents. Their antioxidant properties are needed for cleaning up toxins and harmful by-products that are produced through stresses to our body. They also provide fibre and moisture to keep the digestive system functioning efficiently. When eaten raw, they provide the life-giving enzymes that fire off many chemical reactions needed for the body's functions.

Fruits and vegetables are also alkalising, or balance the pH of your body. The pH is a measure of the acidity of the blood tissue in the body. It's measured as acid or alkaline and can be in the range of 1 to 14, with 7.35 being the optimal balance. If the pH level in the blood becomes too acidic, the blood becomes deprived of oxygen causing disease and organ damage to occur.

The body works really hard to maintain an optimal pH level. This requires a lot of energy. If the body has to work doubly hard to balance its pH then stresses are placed on how the body functions efficiently. Acidic foods and drinks invite illness and a lack of energy while alkaline foods promote good health and the easy elimination of toxins.

To increase the amount of fruits and vegetables in your diet, aim to choose as many different coloured fruits and vegetables as possible to ensure that you have a wide range of vitamins and minerals occurring naturally in your food plans.

Other plant foods to include are almonds, walnuts, Brazil nuts, sunflower seeds, sesame seeds, pumpkin seeds, linseed, beans, small amounts of grain in the form of rolled oats, quinoa, basmati rice, spelt flour, wholegrain bread and small amounts of sun-dried fruit such as raisins, currants, sultanas, prunes and apricots.

Another way of incorporating plant foods is to use fresh herbs to flavour cooked food and salads. Dried herbs can be also be used in teas for elemental nutritional benefit. An example is liquorice root and peppermint tea, which support digestive functions.

What's interesting is that nuts and seeds fulfill three daily requirements because they have protein, essential fatty acids, fibre and, in the case of sesame seeds, calcium.

LOW GLYCAEMIC INDEX CARBOHYDRATES

The Glycaemic Index (GI) is a measurement of how fast the carbohydrate of a food enters your bloodstream resulting in a boost in blood sugar levels. When you constantly eat foods with a high GI, your blood sugar levels rise very quickly – as does your energy level. With high GI foods your blood sugar level plummets just as quickly, leaving you tired and craving more sugary carbohydrates for an instant energy hit.

Foods that cause a rapid rise in blood sugar levels can also cause inflammation and a sudden rise in insulin levels, which places stress on your body. This up and down release of insulin levels can deplete your stores of insulin and become a precursor for type 2 diabetes.

High GI foods include sugar, potatoes, breads made from refined flour, pastries and cakes, corn and potato chips, soft drink (soda) and sweets; that is, mostly refined and pre-packaged foods. If you want to follow a low GI diet or find out more information on GI foods, it is best to get a resource book. It will give you more detailed information on what foods are high and low GI and provide a comprehensive list of low and high GI values so that you can make your food choices accordingly.

Low GI foods to include in your diet:
• wholegrain breads
• natural muesli (to replace processed breakfast cereals)
• egg pasta made from durum wheat or spelt
• spelt flour which has a high protein content
• legumes and pulses
• basmati rice or quinoa
• pumpkin or sweet potato (instead of potato)
• cakes made from almond meal instead of white flour.

Learning how to create meals with a balanced approach to the GI means you choose mostly low GI foods in your daily food intake. The slow absorption from low GI carbohydrates means that you get a steady flow of energy. You will feel more balanced and put less stress on your pancreas.

ESSENTIAL FATTY ACIDS – THE GOOD FATS

Many people think that all fat is bad for your health. Eating a low-fat diet is hard to maintain because low-fat foods just don't satisfy. Good fat provides a concentrated source of energy in the diet and also satisfies the appetite. Eating the right kind of fat is essential to life. Many of your body's tissues rely on its insulating effect. More than 70 per cent of your brain and nerve cells are made up of fat. Fats help in the absorption of fat-soluble vitamins, which may not be absorbed if there's no fat.

However, there are good fats and bad fats. The good fats help prevent clogging of the arteries and lower bad cholesterol. Good fat will also moisten your digestive system. Many people have approached me at events to comment on how efficient their digestive system has become when they have introduced essential fatty acids into their meals. A simple way to do this is to have pesto with cold-pressed extra virgin olive oil and it's really easy to make (see recipe on p98). Cold-pressed oil is the best choice because the oil is extracted from the olives without the process of adding heat. When oil is heated to high temperatures its health benefits diminish.

Good fats to include in your diet:

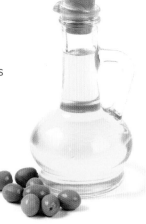

- cold-pressed extra virgin olive oil
- avocados
- almonds
- walnuts
- macadamia nuts
- Brazil nuts
- pecan nuts
- sesame seeds
- linseeds
- tahini
- sunflower seeds
- pumpkin seeds
- oily fish (such as sardines, salmon, mackerel, tuna and fish oil supplements).

Bad fats are mostly solid at room temperature and basically clog up your arteries, increasing your risk of heart disease. The more processed a fat, the harder it is to digest. Avoid overheating fat as deep frying or burning fat changes its nature, making it harder for your body to digest. Other bad fats are trans fats, which are highly processed fats and are commonly found in processed foods.

Fats to avoid or minimise include:

- butter
- highly processed cheese
- cream cheese
- sour cream
- camembert
- brie
- ice-cream
- cream
- lard
- sausages
- skin on poultry
- bacon
- blended vegetable oils
- highly processed vegetable spreads
- fatty cuts of red meat
- fried food.

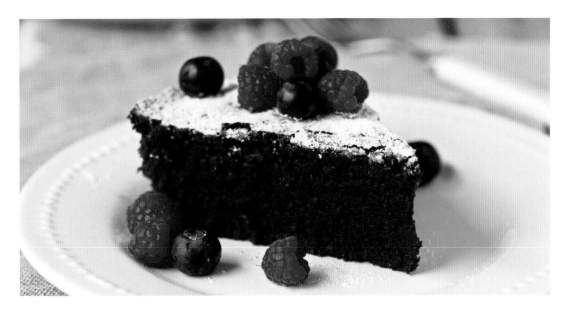

TREATS

There are many reasons why sugar is of no benefit to your health. However the front tip of your tongue is the area that responds to sweet tastes and not having a sweet finish to a meal may leave you feeling unsatisfied. You may choose to completely remove sugar from your diet, but for many people this is unrealistic. It may lead to bingeing on these sweet treats instead. Plus, labelling treats as 'bad' or 'no-no's' sets up a pattern of denial and increases the craving that people will have for sweet foods.

I really like to treat myself and the thought of giving up chocolate altogether, or not sharing a cake with friends, does not appeal. Replacing nourishing meals with these foods is not a healthy strategy either. So I realised that if I replaced bingeing on these foods with an occasional treat, it actually became a pleasure. Instead of overdoing my favourite sweets, they are now something I look forward to and savour slowly. What I also found was that when I have nourishing meals, I don't crave sweets for energy.

An occasional sweet treat is now a delight rather than a choice that leaves me feeling guilty.

Look for treats that have some nourishing ingredients like fruit, almond meal or ricotta. In this way you will find the treat is nourishing and filling and you won't eat too much of it. It's fine to have a treat that is not recommended in a healthy diet, just don't eat too much of it and always return to the blueprint of *The Metabolic Clock* program.

Examples of treats include:

- good quality chocolate in small amounts (not the whole block!)
- fresh figs and dates
- liquorice
- almond friands
- poached fruit with natural yoghurt
- baked ricotta cake
- flourless chocolate cake
- muesli slice
- sorbet and soy ice-cream

Natural activities that feed your life force

As well as the five categories of food that I include in my diet every day I also ensure that I include natural activities that feed my life force.

FEEDING YOUR LIFE FORCE

Do you ever have the feeling that you need to get out of the city and spend some time in the country to reconnect with nature? Why wait? You can do some simple things every day that reconnect you with the energy of nature. Most of these activities are very simple and in natural abundance.

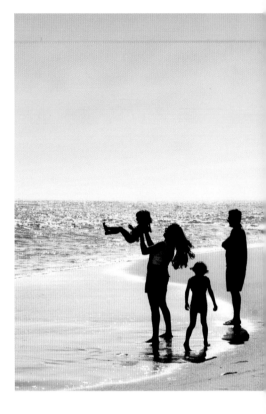

- Go for a walk along the beach, in a forest, or a park.
- Sit quietly in the early morning sun.
- Find something funny to laugh at; see a funny movie; read a funny book; or go to a comedy show.
- Smile at everything. It may feel awkward at first, but you will soon enjoy it.
- Drink water.
- Eat a raw salad every day.
- Learn to meditate.
- Think about what you are grateful for every day.
- Move your body, go for a walk, swim, jog, cycle, skip, and dance or play sport.
- Eat two pieces of fruit every day.
- Give an act of kindness: it's an instant way to feel good about yourself.
- Watch the sun rise. Watch the sun set.
- Eat lots of green plant food.
- Take long, deep breaths often.
- Have a cup of boiled water with freshly squeezed lemon juice every morning.

Creating a daily routine that nourishes and heals

When creating your daily routine, eat most of your food throughout the day. Kick-start your metabolism by eating an early breakfast, keep it moving with mid-morning fruit, fuel it along with a midday meal, add a small protein snack mid-afternoon and eat a protein and enzyme-rich meal early in the evening. Have a small treat, then stop eating and relax to prepare for healing sleep. If you go to bed feeling light, your metabolism will relax and energy will be available for your body's healing processes while you sleep.

When you align yourself with the natural energy cycles of The Metabolic Clock *you will feel empowered to make healthy lifestyle changes.*

Food supplements that support natural weight loss

Diagnostic testing by a health specialist is recommended to identify what you specifically require, however, the following supplements generally boost an individual's health and support natural weight loss.

GREEN BARLEY POWDER
The green grass of barley sprouts is juiced and then dried to produce green barley powder. It is a convenient nutritional supplement that is packed with nourishment. You would have to eat a massive plate of green vegetables to come close to the nutrition that is packed into a teaspoon of green barley powder. It provides a wide spectrum of nutrients that includes vitamins, minerals, amino acids, proteins, enzymes, chlorophyll and antioxidants. It's also alkalizing to the pH of your blood.

Add a teaspoon of green barley powder to your morning juice to encourage cell growth of hair and nails; your skin will also improve with this added nutrition.

SPIRULINA
Spirulina is a green powder made from fresh water algae and is 70 per cent protein. It's easy to digest and is so nutritious that it acts as an appetite suppressant. It's very alkalizing and feeds the body's beneficial intestinal flora. It also helps to regulate the hormone system because it has substantial amounts of essential fatty acid.

FISH OIL
It's ironic that having fish oil reduces the craving for fatty foods. The essential fatty acids in fish oil alleviate depression and the painful inflammation of rheumatoid arthritis. It lowers blood pressure and reduces bad cholesterol. It prevents plaque from building up on the arterial walls, providing protection from strokes and heart attacks. It also contributes to prevent breast, colon and prostate cancer as well as improving eyesight, skin, hair, nails and teeth.

PROBIOTICS
Probiotics are beneficial live bacteria that are essential in the digestive system to break down the nutrients in food for digestion and assimilation of nutrients. They help digest proteins, carbohydrates and fats. These good bacteria keep the colon healthy and clean while strengthening the immune system and retarding yeast infections.

FIBRE SUPPLEMENT
Fibre helps maintain normal bowel movements. Fibre is beneficial for intestinal bacteria to help maintain healthy digestion. It also promotes elimination and rids the body of waste, having a cleansing effect on the bowel.

ACAI BERRY JUICE
This fruit grows wild in the Amazon rainforests. It's a rich source of protein that satisfies the appetite, making it ideal for weight loss. It contains dietary fibre and has antibacterial properties that improve digestion. The high levels of essential fatty acids play a major role in lowering cholesterol in the blood. Add Acai berry juice to your morning juice.

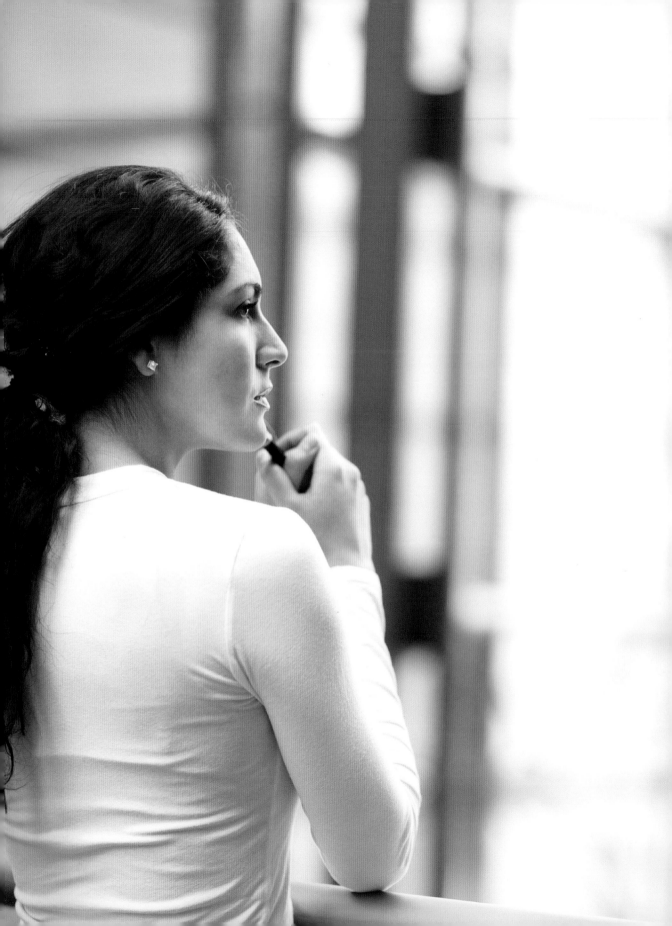

Step 2

How to create the motivation to attain your weight loss and wellness goals

'Life takes on meaning when you become motivated, set goals and charge after them in an unstoppable manner.' – Les Brown

In this section you will learn how to create a healthy thinking strategy that will motivate you to achieve your weight loss and wellness goals. You will also learn how to overcome disempowering thought patterns and create healthy behaviors and practices. Once and for all, you'll feel confident and motivated to maintain a healthy lifestyle.

Have you struggled to sustain your motivation or just to get started with something new? This section is just what you need to make lasting changes to your lifestyle. Your motivation is driven by how you are feeling. Your feelings are a response to what you are thinking. Therefore, what you are thinking will either be the fuel or the extinguisher of your motivation.

There are six ways of thinking that will create the internal motivation to stay focused on making lifestyle changes and attain your weight loss and wellness goals.

1. Start thinking like a healthy person.
2. Create impassioned thinking.
3. Mind sweep to clear out disempowering thoughts.
4. Create an 'I can' attitude.
5. Believe everything is possible.
6. Visualize your success.

Chapter 6

Start thinking like a healthy person

Have you noticed that when things are going well it's easy to balance your life and take good care of yourself? In contrast, when life is challenging, it's much harder to maintain that balance and take care of yourself. In these difficult times it's easy to create a pattern of emotional eating and lose sight of your health goals.

If you fill your mind with negative, defeating thoughts, judgements, assumptions and criticisms, they will weigh you down. You are going to feel unfulfilled emotionally because these are empty emotions. The cycle then begins. Because you feel unfulfilled emotionally you may overeat in a subconscious effort to feel fulfilled. No food will fill you up emotionally.

Addressing unhealthy emotions is the only way to overcome emotional eating.

At age 23, I was a champion 1500-metre track and field athlete. I was awarded a scholarship to the Australian Institute of Sport, but shortly after arriving, I injured my knee and had to stop training for a few months. I felt like a failure and became very miserable. Then I began to binge eat and live my life a little recklessly. My weight ballooned, which was very noticeable against the backdrop of 216 elite athletes. This, of course, compounded my feelings of failure and helplessness.

Once my injury had healed I was back into training. However, I was still carrying a lot of extra weight. I began to skip meals to save on calories. I had sugar cravings and would often replace a meal with a packet of chocolate biscuits. I wasn't hungry for food: I was trying to quench my emotional pain.

With all my unhealthy practices I could not lose weight even though I was running 100 kilometres (62 miles) a week. My body clock had become so out of balance that no amount of exercise made a difference to my weight. I was obsessed with fad diets and became even more unbalanced. Because I was not focused on nourishing my body, I lacked energy and was training way out the back of the pack. I often trained on my own without the support of the training group because I was embarrassed about my weight gain.

What I learned from my experience of gaining weight was that I needed to change the way I thought about myself. I simply needed to stop fighting with myself and change my negative thoughts. I began to speak to myself in a kind and loving way.

Addressing your thinking quickly and easily leads to a body transformation. The way to achieve lasting success is to address the way you think about yourself, the way you feel about yourself and how you nurture and treat your body as a lifelong approach to health and wellbeing.

You create yourself by how you think, which creates how you feel which then leads to how you act and how you treat your physical body. These are the raw materials that you use to create you. If you feel good about yourself you will feel more inclined to nourish and nurture yourself.

Creating wellness and fulfilment is as simple as switching your thinking to what you want to experience, to really place all your attention and focus on what you want to experience, rather than on what you don't. This instantly creates inspired feelings and energises you to act in a more empowered way.

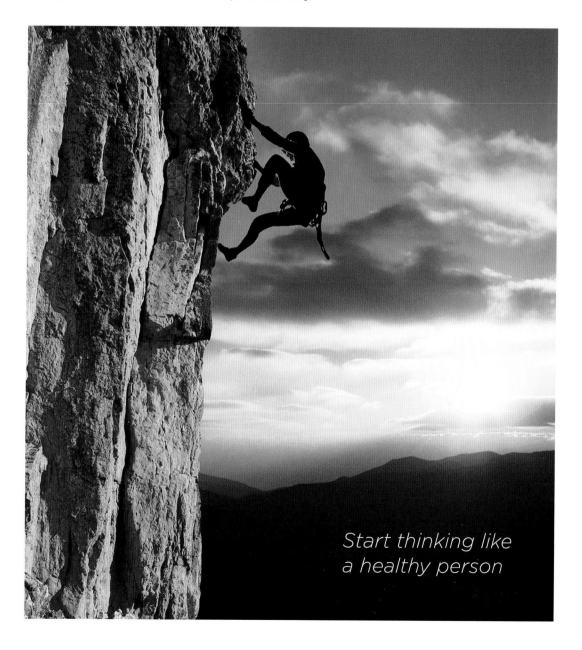

Start thinking like a healthy person

Chapter 7

Create impassioned thinking

There is no nourishment like thinking happy thoughts.

Impassioned thinking has a lot of feeling behind it. Whatever you are thinking creates a feeling in your body, mostly in your gut. Impassioned thinking can be the quickest way to gain energy instantly. Have you ever noticed that you have enthusiasm and energy when you feel passionate about something? This is because your thoughts are a positive match to the thing that you feel passionate about.

Imagine becoming impassioned about creating a healthy lifestyle. Imagine changing your thoughts to match being healthy. This will create good feelings in your body and completely stop emotional eating patterns. Make the decision to be impassioned about being healthy and eating delicious food that nourishes you.

You are the creator of your own experience

This can be a little scary at first because if you don't like the way you have created yourself or if you don't like the life experience that you are having, then it would no longer make sense to blame anyone else. You will no longer be able to blame your parents, your partner, your boss, your friends or your DNA.

Only you know what it's like to be you. Therefore the most important person in your world to listen to is YOU!

In your mind you form opinions about yourself and the world around you. Based upon what you are thinking and the pictures that you see in your mind's eye, your body responds with a feeling or an emotion. These emotions can feel good or bad. Good feelings vitalise you, bad feelings de-vitalise you.

Are your thoughts about yourself kind, or are they unfriendly and destructive? You are going to act out your life based on what you feel. Are you living your best life or are you experiencing your life with self-created demons? Remember, your thoughts can either empower you – or not.

Be aware of what you are thinking about yourself and you will quickly realise this creates how you feel. Learning how to create empowering thoughts will alter how you feel about yourself, which translates to how you treat your body. Your empowering self talk will become the motivational rocket fuel to achieve your outcomes.

THE THINKING YOU
It's how you use your mind to think that creates major transformations in your life quickly and easily. Learning how to stop negative self-talk and speak to yourself in a positive and nurturing way is the quickest way to reshape your body and your life.

THE FEELING YOU

Feelings of joy and enthusiasm empower you to positive action. Feeling threatened, lonely, anxious or stressed can lead to an emotional eating pattern or addiction along with a feeling that you have no control or willpower. By identifying the negative thoughts behind the feeling and reforming them with positive words, you will create more motivation and empowerment. This leads to feeling good about yourself and will help you to avoid triggering unhealthy behaviors.

THE PHYSICAL YOU

Your choices of how you feed your body, how you use it, how you maintain it and how you ask it to respond determine what your body will look like and how comfortable it will feel.

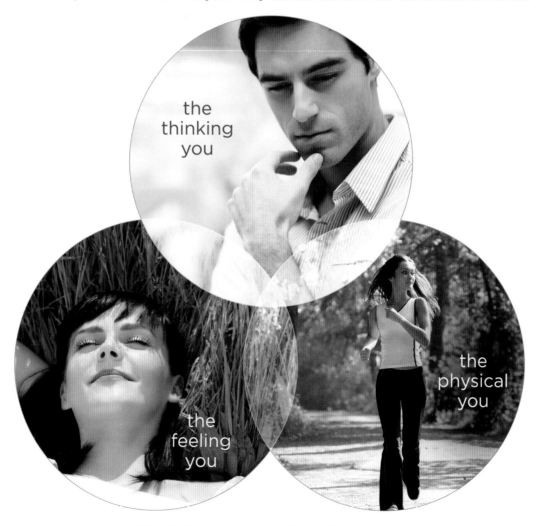

the
thinking
you

the
feeling
you

the
physical
you

The thinking part of you activates the feeling part of you, which determines how the physical part of you will act. It all links up together.

I'm not ready

It always amazes me when I hear, 'I'm not ready', or 'When I'm ready'. For example when a cigarette smoker tells me that he could give up smoking as soon as he decides that he is ready.

I respond with, 'Ready for what, experiencing a major health crisis?'

Are you not ready to live and to thrive? Who doesn't want to experience optimal wellness and fulfilment? The real question is not, 'Are you ready?' but, 'Are you willing?'

Are you willing to have a great body, a healthy heart and lots of vital energy to do the things that you love? Are you willing to do something different in order to get a different result?

It's rare and refreshing to meet people who think wonderfully and joyfully about their lives. I meet many people who spend most of their time thinking about what's not working in their lives, all the things that are wrong in their lives, all the things that need fixing in their lives and constantly complaining about the people in their lives. These types of people are left wondering why their lives aren't bringing them happiness.

It almost seems like a there is a basic instinct to blame, judge and complain, thinking that external factors are the cause of pain and suffering. To add to this, opinions are then created to justify the feeling of having no choice in outcomes. These opinions then become a blueprint of how life will be experienced. Change the opinions and the outlook will change. Don't change and the experience remains the same. These thoughts and opinions lead to giving up on any goals that are being aimed for.

This can also lead to patterns of emotional eating. The thoughts or opinions and the judgements of others, and most of all of yourself, leave you feeling very uncomfortable. With your desire to feel good again you reach out for whatever you think will make you feel good. This could mean a block of chocolate, too much alcohol, high carbohydrate food or simply ignoring the cues that you are full and overeating. The truth is that you actually feel worse with this behaviour and become judgemental of yourself, perpetuating a cycle that seems to control you.

> **Imagine a baby elephant in the circus. The circus owner ties a rope around the ankle of the elephant and stakes the rope to the ground. The baby elephant pulls on it and isn't strong enough to pull it out of the ground. He forms the opinion that he is weak and trapped.**
>
> **When he grows to be an adult he carries this opinion with him – and remains staked to the ground. It may have been true for him as a baby elephant, but as an adult elephant, it's certainly not true. You and I both know that elephants are possibly the strongest animals on earth and as such he could easily pull the stake out of the ground – it's only the opinion that holds the adult elephant back.**

When you were a child, did you listen to people who told you that you had no choice? Did you form opinions in your childhood that you still drag around today? Do they work for you or do they limit you and hold you back? It doesn't matter who told you that you were weak, stupid and chubby or that you were never going to amount to anything. What matters is whether or not you believed them!

What is required is a simple shift of opinion about yourself. A shift in perception in your own mind will automatically change the way you feel about yourself, which will alter how you treat yourself. This then gives control of you back to *you*.

Who creates you?

Your parents may have initially created you, or your belief system tells you that God created you. Who do you think creates you in this present moment? As an adult you create yourself. Take responsibility for how you are creating yourself. If you don't like it, change it. If you decide that your current thinking is not going to move you towards what you want, then change it so that you create what you want instead of what you don't want. You will realize how powerful you are when it is you that starts transforming your own body and life.

Recently I was at my local supermarket checkout waiting to go through. I noticed a popular women's magazine with a picture of an overweight and depressed celebrity on the front. The headline read that she was miserable because she was fat. I began to think about this statement and realised that this statement was incorrect. It should have read, she is fat because she is miserable. Once you identify the negative self-talk that creates your response to miserable feelings, you will be more resourceful and empowered; you will know what you have to change.

If you want to transform yourself, what you say to yourself is the first creative tool that you can use. The second is how you feel when you think these thoughts. The third is what practices and behaviours you choose as a consequence of thinking and feeling this way.

When you understand how you have created yourself, you are in a position of choice. You can continue creating yourself the same way or you can re-opinion your thoughts, which will then alter your feelings about yourself, which will then ultimately change how you treat your body. You will begin to attract and create what you desire instead of what you do not want.

Chapter 8

Mind sweep to clear out disempowering thoughts

Have you heard of the term 'enlightened being'? Consider how you feel when you are happy and joyous. Does this feel light? Now consider how heavy you feel when you are grumpy or sad or depressed or angry or overwhelmed. Do these feelings of heaviness then translate into eating foods that make you heavy? Does this food then weigh you down with body fat? Perhaps an enlightened being thinks light thoughts, creating light feelings. If you would like to lose weight maybe a simple approach is to lighten up by getting rid of those heavy thoughts.

Every thought that you have is going to empower you towards your goals or disempower you, leading to destructive behaviours. Focusing on being fat and thinking about why you are fat and how fat you are, and that you will always be fat is going to make it difficult to act like a healthy, slim person.

What is a mind sweep?

A mind sweep is when you observe your thoughts and really pay attention to what you are thinking. You can then sweep out the repeated negative thoughts that keep cropping up. Write out all your disempowering thoughts you have about yourself. Once you have listed your thoughts you can look at them and decide which ones are useful and which ones need to be swept out.

Empowering thoughts	Disempowering thoughts
• My desire is to be fit and healthy.	• I hate exercising.
• It's time for me to feel more vital.	• I can't stop eating.
• I would like to join a gym.	• I need chocolate.
	• I'm not worthy of success.
	• I'm scared of change.
	• I'm not quite ready.
	• I don't know where to begin.
	• I'm not sure I can do it.

> It's easy to see that the disempowering thoughts far outweigh the empowering thoughts.

This is the way I am, I can't change

I often hear people say, 'This is the way I am, I can't change.' With this type of opinion, how do you expect to transform anything? This sort of opinion will prevent you from getting started on the goals you are aiming for. Create your own empowering opinions to fit your own situation and your own personal goals.

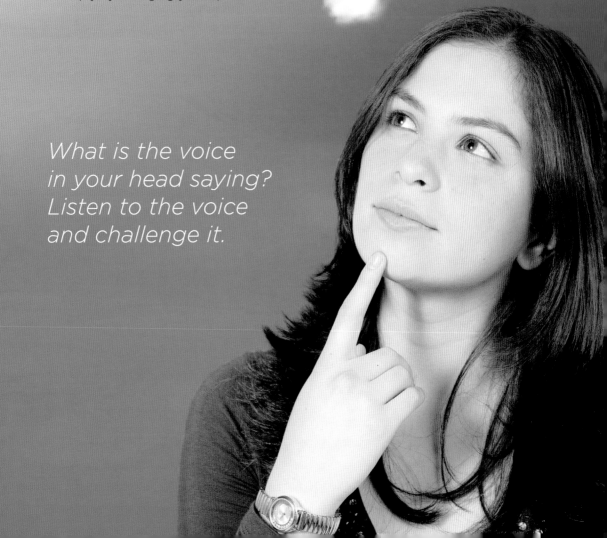

When you were born you were a pure spirit finding your way into a new body. You had to learn how to lie on your back, roll over, crawl and walk. Nobody could do this for you. You learned how to do new things with enthusiasm and a desire for finding out and knowing. The first time you tried to walk you did not give up when you fell over. As you grew up and reached adulthood, slowly something changed within you. You listened to other people's opinions about how to behave and be yourself in this world. This transformed the desire for following your instinct to learned patterns of behaviour. As you were growing up, these learned patterns of behaviour formed the ideas of what you think about yourself today. These patterns of behaviour can be unlearned. The key to this 'unlearning' is that you have to be willing to change them.

The great visionary and teacher Reverend Ike had a simple saying: Whatever you put after 'I am', you become.

We all have lots of 'I ams' that are opinions we have formed about ourselves. They are mini identities that can empower or disempower us. You can shatter disempowering identities simply by changing your opinions.

What is the voice in your head saying? Listen to the voice and challenge it.

Mind sweep to create empowered thinking

The following process can be used to transform any aspect of your life. Body image is often an easy one to start with. Simply begin to focus on your body image. Start to list your disempowering opinions about yourself. Rant and rave and collect all your opinions. When you have collected all these opinions, write down how it makes you feel when you think these thoughts. Then write down how you treat your physical body when you think and feel this way. The more honest you are and the more responsibility you accept for yourself, the quicker you will transform.

An example of mind sweeping

Marion's disempowering opinions about her body image are:

- I am fat.
- I am round and heavy.
- I am chubby.
- I am scared that I will get sick.
- I am stuck.
- I am useless.
- I hate myself.
- I am weak.
- I can't do anything right.
- I'm not good enough.
- I'm powerless.

When Marion thinks this way, she feels:

- resentful of others and jealous of what they have that she doesn't
- inferior and insignificant when she compares herself to others
- overwhelmed and tired with these thoughts
- moody and exhausted when these thoughts consume her thinking.

When Marion thinks and feels this way, she:

- eats lots of cake and chocolate
- hibernates at home and sleeps a lot
- stops going out with friends
- stops nurturing herself
- stops eating nourishing food.

Marion changed her disempowering opinions to the following empowering opinions:

- I am OK.
- I am healthy and strong.
- I love to exercise.
- I explore new things with excitement.
- I can do it.
- I am here to contribute.
- I am courageous.
- I flow with life.
- I plan and prepare.

With these new opinions Marion feels:

- motivated and excited
- vital and energized
- significant and considered
- happier and lighter.

This then leads to the new energizing practices that Marion enjoys including:

- nourishing her body with healthy foods
- going to bed before 10 pm and getting up early
- communicating with friends
- socializing and having fun
- exercising regularly.

STEPS TO YOUR OWN PERSONAL MIND SWEEP

1. Find a quiet place and focus on your opinions about your body. Allow your thoughts to flow. Write down your thoughts about your body image, particularly what you say to yourself about it.
2. For example: 'I am fat, I am ugly, I am stupid, I am sick of being sick, I am round, I am trapped, I am heavy, I am a secret eater.'
3. Now focus on the judgements you make of yourself and write these down too. These are judgements you have as to why you haven't made the progress that you wanted. Do not filter or edit these judgements, write them down as they spring to mind.
4. For example: 'I'm not as good as others; I have no willpower, I can't do anything right, I am worthless, I am not good enough, why can't I get this right?'
5. Ask yourself, 'What do I feel when I think this way?'
6. For example: 'I feel frustrated, I feel anxious, I feel unworthy, I feel lonely, I feel sad, I feel unwanted and I feel tired.'
7. Ask yourself, 'When I think and feel this way, how do I treat my physical body?'
8. For example: 'I overeat, I sleep a lot, I take stimulants, I act moody and angry, I eat too much chocolate, I stay up late at night, I secretly eat late at night.'
9. It's time to recognise that these are just opinions that you have formed, or borrowed from hearing what others say. Ask yourself, 'Is this what I desire to experience in my body?' If the answer is a clear 'no', then re-form new opinions for every opinion that you no longer want. It can be as simple as writing the opposite of your unhealthy opinion. Choose positive language and keep your words simple. See the examples below.

> **I am fat becomes I am slim and healthy**
> **I am ugly becomes I am gorgeous**
> **I am stupid becomes I am smart in my own way**
> **I am trapped becomes I am free to choose**
> **I am a secret eater becomes I eat with balance**
> **I am sick of being sick becomes I am healthy and well**

1. Stand up and read these positive opinions out loud and confidently six times. This is very important as you are engaging more senses when you read, speak and hear. Be convincing. Read them six more times if you feel you need to strengthen your opinions a little more. It's important for you to hear them spoken with certainty. This helps you to feel more energized, more alive and more empowered. Put on some upbeat music and have some fun with this.
2. Write down the positive emotions that you feel after reading out your opinions or write down the opinions that will be experienced as you practice with your empowered positive language.
3. As a result of these newfound positive emotions, what are the practises that you will choose to nurture and nourish your physical body? Write down all your new healthy practices.

You may like to use your journal to work through your personal mind sweep.

It's important to note that these new opinions are not affirmations that you might say a few times a day. These new opinions will become your new internal dialogue that you say to yourself repeatedly. Every time a disempowering opinion creeps into your mind, catch the thought and interrupt it by saying, 'Stop!' You can say this out loud or inside your mind, then quickly replace the old opinion with the new empowering one.

Given the lifetime of negative thoughts that you may have had, be patient with yourself. You may need to practise and, like training a muscle, train your mind to think healthy, empowering thoughts. Initially this may feel a little strange because your mind will want to go back to your old patterns of thinking. Keep practising and you will empower yourself to achieve your chosen outcomes.

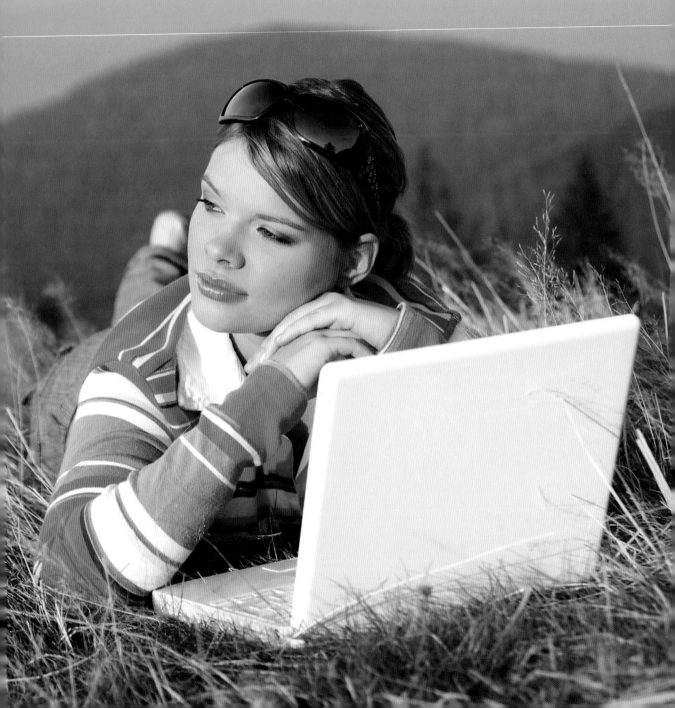

Chapter 9

Create an 'I can' attitude – changing bad habits with three empowering strategies

1 Interrupt unhealthy patterns of thinking

If you turned on your computer and there was a virus file, you wouldn't open the file, wanting to protect your computer. Your instinct would be to delete the rogue file. Think of your mind having 'thought viruses'. These viruses are thought clusters that leave you feeling devitalized and disempowered. These nagging thoughts can whip you into a frenzy, sometimes causing debilitating panic attacks. These thoughts seem real, however; they present false evidence. A 'pattern interrupt' is a quick way to stop these negative thoughts from taking hold.

Imagine sitting with friends in an outdoor café enjoying a conversation. Suddenly a car backfires. In an instant you stop talking and turn your attention towards the car. Your heart could be beating faster if you got a fright. You realise that you are okay, acknowledge the reality of what has happened and turn back to your friends. After this interruption you can't remember what you were talking about so you talk about something else instead. The loud noise created an instant interruption to your pathway of thinking.

You can create an interruption to your thinking when nagging negative thoughts begin to take over in the following way.

- Acknowledge the thoughts that are de-energizing you.
- Say to yourself, 'Stop!'
- Ask yourself, 'Is this what I really want to be thinking?'
- Ask, 'What do I desire? What do I really desire to experience?'
- Switch all your thoughts to opinions that will energise you. Keep persevering until you feel energized.

2 The 5-minute rule

It's your mind that says, 'Have another piece of cake,' not your stomach.

Have you ever felt the overwhelming urge to go back for a second helping of food only to wish that you hadn't because you feel bloated and uncomfortable? Or you are enjoying a piece of cake or some chocolate and it's so delicious that you think that another piece will be just as nice. The thing is, you will probably overdo the treat and feel guilty afterwards. The feeling of guilt causes you to feel bad and to comfort yourself you decide to binge. This is the cycle of emotional eating.

A simple pattern interrupt is the 5-minute rule. When you feel the urge to have another piece of cake, interrupt your thoughts by saying, 'I will wait 5 minutes,' and immediately distract yourself with another activity. Go for a walk, call a friend, put a load of washing on, read a book or clean your car. Chances are that you will forget about that second helping. The urge passes quickly when you create a distraction. What you will gain is a feeling of empowerment with the sense that you are back in control.

When you begin to make lifestyle changes, the first 3 days are the hardest. You may need to create distractions to break the old patterns of behaviour. For example, if you're having alcohol-free nights as one of your outcomes, you may choose to go to a yoga class or the gym at night as a distraction. Think of something else you can do to replace sitting at home with a glass of wine. Once you get through the first three days you have momentum and it begins to get easier.

3 Changing an unhealthy pattern

I am aware of the negativity, but I choose not to dwell on it.

Take charge of the creative control of your mind. Have you ever noticed the relationship between stress and emotional eating? Do you know the triggers that make you want to have a stimulant to get a lift or to eat to get relief from a stressful situation? The following process is about making these connections and knowing the impacts that they have on your life and your vitality. The more consciously you are aware of your responses and what brings them on, the more you can prepare yourself to make healthy choices.

The key to overcoming an unhealthy choice is to learn how to *respond* to a trigger rather than *reacting* to a trigger. Responding means that you are choosing your action. By responding, you can take an unhealthy practice and transform it into a healthy practice.

Your mind is constantly creating solutions for you whether you are aware of it or not. If you are feeling bad, your mind starts searching for something to make you feel good. Your mind associates having alcohol with a happy memory so it presents this as an option for you. You get an idea to have some wine. It might be that your mind associates having chocolate with a happy memory so it suggests that you buy a block of chocolate at the supermarket on your way home from a stressful day.

The most important thing to recognise about unhealthy practices, particularly if they are emotionally driven, is that what you are really seeking is the experience of a good feeling.

For example, if someone has had a stressful and demanding day at work they may come home feeling like they need an alcoholic drink. What they are really seeking is the feeling of relaxation. They may think that alcohol will give them a state of relaxation, however, other practices such as having a massage, taking a bath, walking in the park or meditating are relaxing without being a stimulant.

Recognising what you desire to feel will help widen the choices available to you and your options of how to achieve this positive feeling. Having more choices will open up a range of healthy choices too.

HOW TO CHANGE AN UNHEALTHY BEHAVIOR

1. Choose an unhealthy practice or behavior that you want to change.
2. What is your outcome? Is it to minimise, get rid of, or replace this practice or behavior?
3. Ask yourself, 'Why do I want to change this?' The more compelling the reason, the easier it will be to make a healthy choice.
4. What is the feeling or state of mind that I am really seeking?
5. What healthy practices or behaviors can I choose to create the feeling that I am seeking? Using your imagination and being very resourceful can create many possibilities.
6. When the trigger appears, take a moment to observe your initial reaction. Quickly choose one of your new options for a healthy practice or behavior to create the feeling that you seek at that moment.

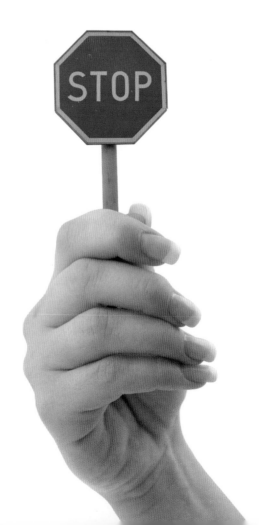

Chapter 10

Believe everything is possible

According to all known laws of aviation there is no way that a bee should be able to fly. Its wings are too small to get its large body off the ground. The bee flies anyway.

When you take action to achieve a goal it does not matter what other people believe, it only matters what you believe.

A very powerful step in any body or life transformation is to believe everything is possible. The repetition of opinions leads to beliefs. Once a belief becomes a deep conviction, things begin to happen.

There are two kinds of beliefs – supportive or unsupportive. Use your imagination to create beliefs that support your transformation. See yourself as you desire to be and believe what you see. You will create all the inspiration and motivation to bring what you see into reality.

Very few people prepare for success. Most people would rather be cautious and choose to be prepared in case of disappointment. They occupy their thoughts with 'What if it doesn't work' and 'If I can't do it, it's because ...' strategies. They justify their opinions of defeat so that there is no disappointment. It's fine to prepare yourself for failure if this is what you wish to experience.

The journey is much more fun if you spend your thoughts on 'What's it going to be like when it works?' or 'What does it feel like to have my dreams and desires become my reality?' If a setback arrives, instead of giving up, observe it, make adjustments to your thinking, and continue to focus on your dreams. Live as though you already have them within your grasp.

Kate Smyth was in her mid-twenties and was 20 kilos (44 lbs) heavier than she is today. Kate was unhappy with the way she felt and wanted to change some of her unhealthy behaviors. She decided to set herself a challenge to run a marathon. She did not mind how long it took because her goal was to run the 42 kilometres (26 miles) without stopping. After completing her first marathon Kate felt so good about herself that she decided to train to run another marathon.

Six years later, Kate qualified to represent Australia in the marathon at the 2006 Melbourne Commonwealth Games and finished in seventh place. Once recovered Kate set a new goal to represent Australia at the 2008 Beijing Olympics and began her training. When I met Kate she only had a few weeks to qualify to be in the Olympic team. Her training had been hampered through illness and the odds were not in favour of her qualifying, however, she believed that she would be in the team.

continued next page

For Kate to achieve her goal she needed to run a personal best time. She set a goal to run 2 hours and 28 minutes for her next marathon. This would leave no doubt in the selectors' minds that she deserved her place in the Olympic team. Each day Kate visualized herself running a marathon in 2 hours and 28 minutes. She created six cards with 2.28 I CAN on them. They were placed on the refrigerator, the food cupboard, a light switch in her hallway, the toilet seat, on her front door and on the steering wheel of her car. This was a great way to maintain focus on her goal. She was creating a vision of her future that helped her to maintain motivation. She also set the alarm on her sports watch to beep at 2.28pm every day. When this alarm went each day, she stopped what she was doing and imagined what she would feel like when she had run the marathon in 2 hours 28 minutes.

This style of visualization builds belief and allowance of the goal being achieved. The feelings of joy and happiness then become your guide and you find all the motivation to keep doing what you need to do to succeed. The more you do this the more joy you will experience. So, essentially you are experiencing the joy of success now, before it even shows up. And you will enjoy the journey.

Kate ran a marathon in Japan on Sunday, 20 April 2008. With each step she said to herself, 'I can, I can, I can' in time with her feet hitting the ground. She said this the whole way so that there was no room for defeating thoughts to enter her mind. Kate ran 2 hours 28 minutes and 51 seconds. She had run close to a five-minute personal best time and had easily qualified for selection in the Olympic team. Kate had discovered that believing in herself was a very powerful strategy for the achievement of her dreams.

I was with Kate one day and someone said to her…'Kate, how do you run a marathon?' Kate replied, 'One step at a time.' Maybe you have something you would like to achieve but think that it's too big and overwhelming. Maybe you can break it into little pieces and just like Kate simply start by believing in yourself and take one step at a time.

Are you ready to allow yourself to be happy and healthy with your perfect body shape? The only reason you do not have the perfect body for you right now is because there is a part of you that believes you can't have it or that you can't make the lifestyle changes needed to help you reach your goals.

Begin by looking at what you currently believe about yourself. Make adjustments to your thinking and bring your beliefs about yourself into alignment with your dreams. Beliefs either support your dreams or they don't. Keep the ones that do and stop using the ones that don't.

If you believe that you have to finish everything that is on your plate … then you will.
If you believe that you hate exercising … then you will always struggle to do it.
If you believe that you don't know where to begin … then you will procrastinate and find it difficult to start things.
If you believe that you are not worthy … then you will easily give up.
If you believe that you are not ready … then you stay stuck in a rut.

Your beliefs about yourself will either create motivation for you or they will de-motivate you. Write out a list of your disempowering beliefs and challenge them with new information.

Some examples:

I was taught that I have to finish everything on my plate.

I do not have to finish everything on my plate. When my stomach tells me it's full then that is the right time for me to stop eating.

I hate exercising.

I enjoy exercising because it's an instant way to change how I feel and it's fun.

I don't know where to begin.

I know it's possible to get started. I just take one small step at a time.

I am not worthy.

I am worthy. I want to make the most of the precious gift of my life.

I am not ready.

I am ready for this. I want to enjoy my body and live a happy and healthy life.

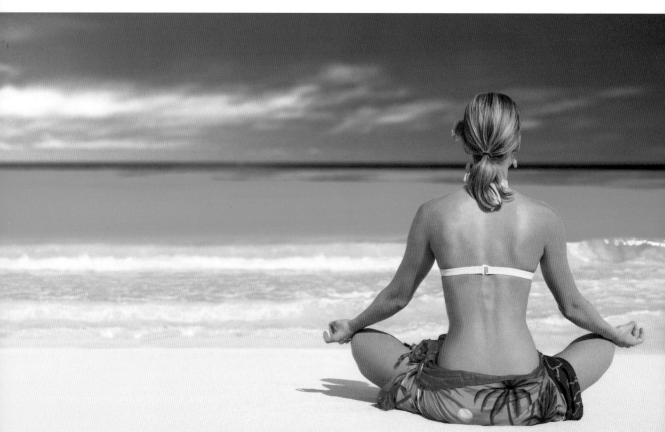

Chapter 11

Visualize your success

*Having mastery over your mind allows
you to have mastery over your body.*

Your body follows your mind. What happens when you decide to get out of bed in the morning? Your body gets up. What happens when you decide you want something to eat? Your body takes you into the kitchen. What happens when you start thinking of being outside when you are in a boring meeting? Your head turns to look outside.

Your body does exactly what you are thinking. It is your servant, not your master. Your body doesn't know the difference between what is real or imagined. Try telling a child who has just had a nightmare that the monster they just saw in their room is not real. Consciously choosing your thoughts will improve the quality of your life.

When you wake up, what are the first thoughts that are on your mind? Are your thoughts compelling enough to propel you out of bed, or are your first thoughts of troubles and problems and all the things that you feel you should be doing that day? Are your thoughts dragging you down and making it hard to get out of bed?

You have an imagination, remember to use it.

Create the practice of morning visualisation. I call it dreaming up your life.

Get up early, sit quietly and direct your thoughts towards how you would like your life to unfold. Use your imagination to create the thoughts and pictures in your mind of all the things that you desire to experience.

Visualisation is more successful when you are relaxed. Three minutes of focused thought at this time is very powerful and provided you only visualise what you desire, you will create a powerful perspective that will make you feel very good.

What is important here is to think only about what you desire. If unwanted thoughts creep in, ignore them by saying 'not now', or 'go away'. Quickly replace them with an empowering thought. This highly energised way of thinking will inspire. See yourself as slim and healthy. See yourself moving your body in a comfortable way. See yourself doing things that you never thought were possible. See yourself being admired and respected. See yourself happy and joyous.

It's just 3 minutes a day to retrain your mind and redirect your life.

This is also a good time to use any empowering language you have created as a result of doing mind sweeps, such as:

- I enjoy eating nourishing food.
- I enjoy being fit and strong.
- I am healthy.
- I am loved and adored.
- I have lots of energy.
- I feel great when I exercise.

There are 86,400 seconds in a day. Three minutes, or 180 seconds, is a very small space of time to dedicate to the happy and healthy vision of your future.

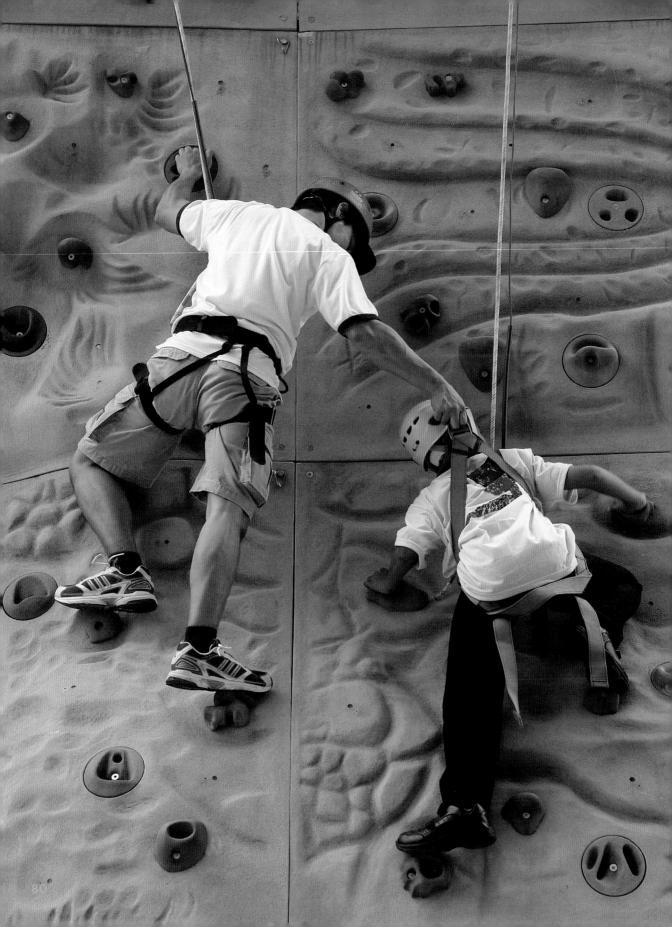

Step 3

How to get started and gain momentum

'Life is like riding a bicycle. To keep your balance you must keep moving.' – Albert Einstein

This section is about overcoming procrastination and creating an action plan that will help you get started. You will learn how to set up a healthy kitchen and discover how easy it is to prepare meals that will nourish you and speed up your metabolism.

Chapter 12

Plan for success

When you are feeling overwhelmed that a goal is too big or too hard to attain, you will probably start procrastinating and may turn to comfort eating to alleviate that uncomfortable feeling. What you really need to do is to stop procrastinating and enjoy the success of gaining momentum for your goal or task ahead. By taking a major goal and breaking it into smaller pieces, it starts to become more approachable and achievable.

Chunking

Chunking is about transforming something that appears overwhelming and impossible into smaller pieces so that it becomes easier and possible. Each goal is made up of pieces – information to find out about, resources to create and action steps to be taken.

The mind can remember things easily in chunks of 9. When there are over nine pieces of information the mind becomes easily confused, lacks focus and becomes overwhelmed. When overwhelmed, it slows or even stalls. Take the goal or task ahead of you and break it into smaller chunks of no more than nine pieces. You will find that the project or task doesn't feel so overwhelming.

Chunking has become a very valuable tool that I use to manage my busy life. When I notice the first signs of overwhelm and procrastination, I stop what I am doing and ask myself, 'How can I break this into smaller pieces?' Once I have chunked the task into smaller pieces, I then choose one small piece to start with.

To overcome procrastination, practise chunking. List one thing that you have been procrastinating about that has prevented you from getting started, and then chunk it into smaller pieces.

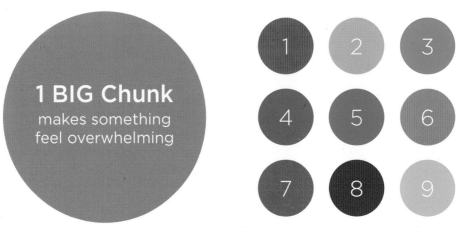

Chunking in action

9 small chunks makes the achievement of a major outcome much easier than 1 BIG Chunk

For example, 'I just can't get motivated to exercise,' chunked into 9 or fewer smaller pieces becomes:

1. Make an appointment with myself to go for a walk.
2. Find myself an exercise buddy.
3. Research sporting facilities and fitness classes in my area.
4. Interview personal trainers.
5. Create compelling reasons to begin exercising.

SEQUENCING

There is an order to the actioning of any chunks. For example, putting your shoes on is more effective if the socks go on first or hosting a party is more successful if the invitations are sent out before the event. Once you have created the key chunks for your outcome, list them in the sequence or order that they need to be done to help you complete the bigger picture.

SORTING

Once you have chunked and sequenced your project, you can sort any information, ideas, things to do and actions to take into the appropriate pieces. Knowing that things are sorted correctly means that you only need to focus on one piece at a time, allowing you to give this part of the project your full attention.

Planning and preparation

If there is one practice that really distinguishes people who create major results in their lives from those who just make it through, it would have to be planning and preparation. Planning and preparation is a powerful strategy that will save you time and money. If you don't create your own strategy for achieving what you desire, then chances are you will fit into someone else's strategy – and that may not lead you to your desired outcome.

If you have planned what you are having for an evening meal before you leave for work, then you will feel less stressed when you are travelling home from work, tired at the end of the day. If you are driving home from work without a plan for your evening meal, the chances are that takeaway food will be very appealing in terms of saving time.

Some ideas to help you plan and prepare

- Allow time for planning and preparation.
- Plan your meals weekly.
- Shop with a list.
- Before starting any new task, spend a few moments thinking about why it's important to you, and then visualize the task as finished. Acknowledge what this feels like.
- Ask yourself, 'Who can add support?'
- Work with a things-to-do list.
- Prioritize and order your list.
- If a task seems too large, chunk it into smaller pieces, then sequence and sort the pieces of information.

Chapter 13

Clean out your cupboards

Do you have clutter in your cupboards? Is your garage messy and full of items needing repair? Is your bookkeeping up to date? Do you keep unwanted items because you think it's wasteful to discard them? Do you keep clothes that you have not worn in years? Are your kitchen cupboards full of expired food or foods that you don't even eat? Are your cupboards so full of clutter that if you opened them, everything would fall out on top of you?

Do you walk around the house saying, 'One day I'll clean out the garage,' or, 'I must get to that cupboard and clean it out, but I just can't cope right now'? Chances are that if your cupboards are cluttered, so are your thoughts.

Are you carrying around old stale thoughts about what you don't want instead of recognising that you do not need those things anymore?

It's time to make way for the new by cleaning out the old.

When we moved to our mountain retreat I had things in boxes for several months because I was too overwhelmed to finish unpacking. I often couldn't find what I was looking for and had no system of organisation. This continued for several months until a very hot summer's day changed the way that I looked at my possessions.

At about 10 am I smelled smoke and looked outside to see plumes of black smoke coming from the forest surrounding the retreat. Within minutes, the fire alarms were sounding and spotter planes were in the air. The Dandenong Ranges were surrounded by three fire fronts gobbling up the dry vegetation.

For the next 5 hours we were on high alert preparing our property for the onslaught of a fire front. In the late afternoon, the police evacuated us from the property fearing that the fire front was very close. We grabbed our pets and some photos and followed the police in our car to a safe exit off the mountain. Looking back, I wondered if my home and all our possessions would be burnt completely. In this moment I realised that all the things that really mattered to me were in the car. My family and my pets were all that I needed. I started to think that I would not need to empty all the boxes anymore and I felt really free.

The following morning, we drove up the mountain through the blackened and burnt forest. Courageously, the volunteer fire fighters had stopped the fire from spreading to the mountain ridge and our home. Our house and those boxes were still there. And I found I was empowered to deal with them by facing the question, 'Do I really need all this stuff?' The answer was no. It was time to get the clean-up started.

You'll be amazed at how much clarity you will gain by deciding to clean out the old. It doesn't matter whether you are storing items because they hold a memory or that you think that one day you may need it. What matters is that energy is required from you to keep these items. They take up space in your cupboards and in your mind. They may also keep you thinking about the past or the future and keep your attention from experiencing the energy of now.

If you are holding on to an item because it holds a special memory for you, then you are holding your thoughts in the past. If you are keeping an item because you think that someday you might need it, then you are sending your thoughts to the future. The most empowering place for your thoughts is in the present and the now.

A great way to begin is to make a list of all the clean-up projects that you require in your home and work environment. From this list you can create an action plan for the clean-up. Then chunk it into small tasks to make the clean-up easier to tackle.

When I decided to clean out all my cupboards, I made five lists:

1. Sell it.
2. Fix it.
3. Throw it.
4. Give it.
5. Do it.

When I did this exercise several years ago I had quite a large list. I had spent a lot of time blaming, judging and complaining about why I did not have the time or energy to get my life organised. I would feel overwhelmed and then procrastinate. I would then make an unhealthy choice of how to treat my body. I was always trying to find things and I often lashed out angrily at anyone who got in my way. This included the people I loved the most. I recognised that my family deserved a healthier attitude from me, and if I spent half as much time actually cleaning out my cupboards as I did thinking about it, then I would have an organised life quite quickly.

What surprised me was that once I got started, the momentum grew and I had huge resources of energy that drove me to complete all the clean-ups. I was like a woman possessed, making clear decisions about what I wanted to keep and what I wanted to discard. It seemed that the more I discarded the more opportunities for newness and joy came into my life and my old feelings of being overwhelmed dissolved. Old, frustrating thoughts that I used to have also disappeared. I began to notice that when I had these thoughts my energy levels dropped.

What do you say about your environment and how does it make you feel? If it's not vital and empowering, maybe it's time to clean out your cupboards.

Enjoy the feeling of satisfaction and achievement to be gained by cleaning out your cupboards and feel the boost in vitality. Choose a cupboard to be cleaned up and take everything out. Look at the clean empty space and put back the things you really need. Give away, donate to a charity or throw away the rest. One cupboard done, you can work your way through the others by breaking up the task into smaller chunks.

Chapter 14

Inspire yourself to achieve with a 21-Day Lifestyle Challenge

I used to be very good at identifying goals for my life, but getting started was very difficult. I often felt overwhelmed at the task that stretched out before me.

Achieving any goal is a step-by-step process of making decisions and taking action. The first decision is to start.

Would you like to burn off more than 20 kilos (44 lbs) of body fat but are worried that it's a big task and it's going to take a long time? These thoughts may overwhelm you and make it difficult to get started. Instead, use the 21-Day Lifestyle Challenge to chunk your weight loss goal into smaller pieces. This will enable you to focus for just 21 days on the practices that will get you started. At the completion of 21 days you will have momentum and can make adjustments to your action plan.

With the use of many 21-Day Lifestyle Challenges you will be able to reach your weight loss and wellness goals.

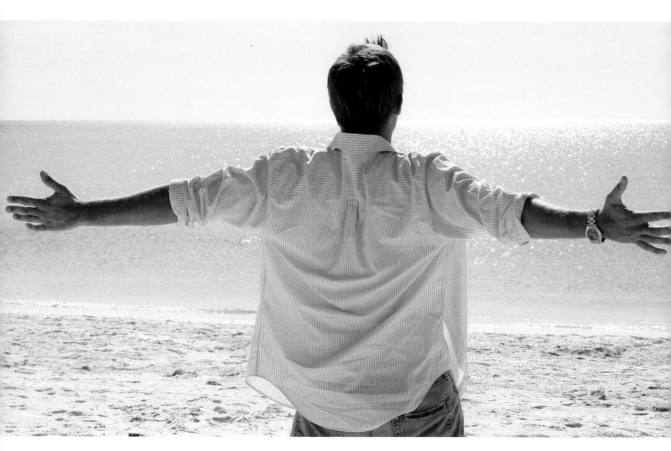

Gain momentum towards creating the life you desire

When you have momentum, everything becomes easier and more achievable. When starting a new lifestyle challenge, the first three to four days take the most effort. By the fourth or fifth day of the challenge, it becomes a little easier and more enjoyable.

In those first few days, you may need to distract yourself from the old pattern of behaviour; replace it with something else or apply the 5-Minute Rule (see p73). This will help break the behaviour cycle. For example if your usual behaviour is to nibble snack food after your evening meal you could create a new behaviour of walking the dog at this time or going to a yoga or dance class instead of sitting on the sofa.

Doing the challenge allows you to focus for 21 days on the practices that you want to change or adopt. It doesn't matter how many times you get it right. What matters is how much momentum you gather along the way towards achieving your outcome. You can set a new lifestyle challenge with the outcome of gaining even more momentum.

Along your challenge journey, an old pattern or obstacle may present itself which impacts on your momentum. See this as an opportunity in disguise. They are probably the things that have held you back in the past and need to be addressed to allow you to move forward. This is where you can identify unhealthy patterns of thinking and replace them with positive language.

Creating your 21-Day Lifestyle Challenge

1. Decide what your goal is.
2. List the reasons it's important to you.
3. Decide on the specific practices or behaviors that you need to do to realize your outcome. (Choose only up to six so that you are not going to feel overwhelmed.)
4. Write down what your reward will be for reaching the 21 days and gaining the vital momentum towards your outcome. Make it worthwhile, as it will become part of your motivation to complete the challenge. If you find yourself presented with an obstacle, the thought of this reward could be the factor that pushes you to complete the challenge. Rewarding yourself in a nurturing way can also become a compelling reason for completing your lifestyle challenge. These rewards can take the form of the following.
   • Enjoy a dinner with someone special.
   • Book a relaxing treatment at a day spa or a pampering weekend away.
   • Play a game of golf.
   • Shop for some new clothes.
   • Get a new hairstyle.
   • Book a holiday.
   • Go to the movies.
5. Choose your support team. This is an optional step but it can be a valuable one. It is great to have a buddy or someone alongside you to share experiences and ideas. If you don't know anyone who is on a challenge, find a friend or relative who is a positive support to you and ask him or her for encouragement and support for your challenge.

Look at your 21-Day Lifestyle Challenge every morning for 21 days as a reminder of what you would like to achieve every day. At the end of each day, check off the practices that you completed for the day. I put mine on the refrigerator door.

At the completion of your 21-Day Lifestyle Challenge, take a moment to think about the changes you have made. How much momentum have you created? What worked for you and what can you do differently? It can take many 21-Day Lifestyle Challenges to achieve your outcome. What is really important is to recognise how much momentum you gain with each challenge. The progress and adjustments you have made will help you to achieve your weight loss and wellness goals.

If you go off track, don't judge yourself. Think about your compelling reasons to make healthy lifestyle changes and create a new 21-Day Lifestyle Challenge. This will help you focus and keep the momentum.

21-Day LIfestyle Challenge

Date: 1st March to the 21st March

Desired practices	1	2	3	4	5	6	7	8	9	10	11	12	13	14	15	16	17	18	19	20	21
1 Eat breakfast every day	✓		✓		✓		✓	✓		✓			✓		✓			✓			✓
2 2 pieces of fruit mid-morning		✓			✓			✓		✓	✓		✓		✓			✓			
3 Eat carbs only during the day	✓		✓				✓		✓			✓			✓	✓			✓		
4 Eat a salad every day	✓	✓		✓		✓		✓			✓		✓			✓	✓				✓
5 Be in bed by 10.30 pm	✓				✓		✓		✓			✓			✓		✓				
6 Go for a 30 minute walk	✓		✓		✓					✓					✓			✓		✓	

Goal	Why is it important to me?	My reward	My support team
To create a healthy routine and balance my metabolic clock. To feel more energised.	I want to overcome some unhealthy habits. I want to live more naturally and look more healthy.	A visit to a day spa that I have always wanted to go to. Might take a friend.	My best friend Jeannette. My partner. This will be good for them to.

The basic principles of
The Metabolic Clock

1. Create compelling reasons to change your lifestyle. You need to decide why you would like to be healthy and enjoy a slim comfortable body.
2. Your metabolism is the engine room of your body. It processes the food you eat, absorbs the nutrients and converts them into fuel, then eliminates waste. It also houses 70 per cent of your immune system, which is your body's first line of defence from foreign invaders.
3. Eat breakfast early in the morning to give your metabolism a kick-start.
4. If you don't eat carbohydrates at night you will burn body fat while you sleep. The role of carbohydrates is to provide energy. You don't need much energy to sleep, so if you eat carbohydrates at night your body will store this energy as fat while you sleep. If you go to bed without eating carbohydrates then the reverse will happen and your body will burn your body fat for energy while you sleep.
5. Get some before midnight sleep. Before midnight sleep helps your body to heal and burn body fat. This also assists in creating balance between the two appetite-regulating hormones, ghrelin and leptin.
6. Eat your food slowly and chew thoroughly before swallowing. Give your attention to what you are eating. Always sit down to eat and ensure that you eat in a relaxing environment.
7. Eat a large raw salad every day. Raw salad vegetables are very low in calories so you can eat plenty of them. When you eat a big salad there is a large volume of fibre to work its way through your digestive system, providing a workout for your colon. In other words, this is 'the exercise program that doesn't raise a sweat'. The enzymes in raw food act like spark plugs to fire up many healing processes within your body.
8. Eat fruit mid-morning. As the sun continues to rise and gain momentum, so too does your metabolism. The Metabolic Clock starts speeding up around 10 am, so a fruit meal at this time will process very quickly. Fruit processes in your digestive system faster than any other food so eating fruit mid-morning is really going to speed up your metabolism.
9. Moving your body or exercising is vital if you approach it firstly to feel good and then to look good. Exercising is a method to disperse negative emotions and to quickly create vital energy. It's quite simple: exercise to feel good about yourself. You will speed up your metabolism because exercise increases your basal metabolic rate.
10. Eat food in its most natural state. Fresh food has energy or a life force that is not present in packaged or processed food. Eat smaller amounts of food more often.
11. Have a cup of boiled water with fresh lemon juice every day as a detox. Lemon juice turns to alkaline in your digestive system balancing high acidity levels.
12. Every thought you think creates a chemical reaction in your body that energizes or de-energizes you. Turn your negative thoughts about yourself into empowering self-talk.
13. Plan your healthy lifestyle. Create 21-Day Lifestyle Challenges to create the motivation to make healthy lifestyle changes.

Chapter 15

Getting your Metabolic Clock kitchen organized and planning your meals

Planning and preparation make it easier to eat nourishing and flavourful foods. This will enable you to easily burn body fat while maintaining high levels of energy. Decide to become passionate about healthy food: this will help make preparing nourishing meals interesting.

As a busy working mother, I quickly learned that if I didn't have a food plan each morning for the family's meals for the day, we often ate takeaway for dinner. If you don't make a plan for your meals then chances are that you will fit into someone else's plans and this is probably going to be a takeaway restaurant's plan for you to eat an unhealthy meal. Creating daily and weekly food strategies will take the guesswork out of your day and help you to relax at mealtimes.

The following food strategies will:

• save you time and money
• assist you to reach your weight loss outcome more quickly
• make it easier for you to be committed to yourself
• increase your energy
• have you looking and feeling younger
• prevent impulsive eating from occurring
• empower you.

Strategies to create organization

Some people say that the desire to eat begins with the eyes. If you make your food look inviting, your eyes will send messages to your brain, triggering your mouth to salivate, awakening the taste buds. A big part of the enjoyment of going out to dinner is to see how creatively a chef presents your food. They know that your eating experience is not measured by taste alone. You may not be a chef, but you can use some of their techniques in your own kitchen.

• Put some creativity into how you present your meals.
• Collect healthy recipes from magazines and cookbooks.
• Clean out your kitchen cupboards. Eliminate clutter and discard stale, out-of-date foods and unhealthy snack foods.
• Stock your pantry with nourishing ingredients that form the basis for many healthy meals. This also adds variety.
• Prepare ahead. Make nourishing takeaway from home and freeze it, so that you are prepared for busy times. When you have a busy day, remember to take a pre-made meal out of the freezer in the morning. This is actually a lot quicker than waiting for takeaway food to be prepared.
• Plan weekly meals. A preparation plan for your meals will help you to be organized

for busy days. Make a weekly plan from the recipes that you have collected. Creating a weekly menu saves you time and money and avoids the pressure of last minute decisions about what you are going to eat.

- Do not go food shopping on an empty stomach. Your mind will get very excited if you are in a supermarket while hungry and you will find yourself grabbing a salty or sugary snack just to tide you over. You may also notice when you unpack the shopping that quite a few unhealthy foods have made their way into your shopping bags. Eat before you go shopping.

The Metabolic Clock pantry

When you have a pantry well stocked with healthy, nourishing ingredients you will feel confident that you can prepare delicious food. To help you feel prepared in your kitchen, there are two categories in a Metabolic Clock pantry.

- Basic pantry shopping list – these are the foods that are common to many recipes.
- Fresh food shopping list – these are the fresh foods for the recipes that you are choosing each week.

To make shopping easy, make a list of the basic foods that are common to The Metabolic Clock recipes that you enjoy. Each week, as you run out of items from this list, put it on your shopping list. The first time you do this you may have a long shopping list. It's a very rewarding experience to clean out your cupboards of the old unhealthy foods and then replace them with food that is full of nourishment. If you keep stock of all the items on the Basic Pantry list then you simply need to add fresh ingredients and you can create any of the following recipes with a minimum of planning.

Decide what day is shopping day and make your meal selections for the coming week. Check the list of ingredients in the recipes against what's in your pantry, then make a shopping list of what is required and add a fresh food shopping list. Make a preparation schedule and make some recipes at the beginning of the week to save you time during the week.

See the sample shopping list and meal planner form on the following pages.

The pantry form and seasonal produce form relate to all of the recipes in this book.
You can create your own electronic spreadsheets if you would like to add other ingredients.

HOW TO USE THE WEEKLY MEAL PLANNER

Allow some time once a week to fill out your weekly meal planner. I like to do mine on shopping day. I look at my recipes and list all the meals that I would like to eat for the coming week. I match the meals to the seasons. Buying seasonal produce is cheaper and matches the weather. I eat berries in summer and citrus fruits and pears in winter. Then I make a pantry list of the ingredients I need and also a fresh food shopping list. This makes shopping easy.

Basic pantry shopping list

- [ ] almonds
- [ ] almond meal
- [ ] apple juice, organic
- [ ] apricots, dried
- [ ] baking powder
- [ ] barley, green powder
- [ ] barley
- [ ] basmati rice
- [ ] bay leaves
- [ ] brazil nuts
- [ ] black olives
- [ ] butter beans, tin
- [ ] chickpeas, tin
- [ ] cannellini beans, dried
- [ ] Celtic sea salt
- [ ] chapatti bread (store in freezer)
- [ ] chickpeas, dried
- [ ] chilli, dried
- [ ] chocolate, dark
- [ ] chocolate, dark cooking
- [ ] cocoa powder
- [ ] coriander, ground
- [ ] cumin, ground

- [ ] currants
- [ ] dates, dried
- [ ] dijon mustard
- [ ] dry white wine
- [ ] figs
- [ ] fruit spread
- [ ] garam masala
- [ ] gherkins
- [ ] grape seed oil
- [ ] honey (cold extracted)
- [ ] ice-cream cones, plain
- [ ] kidney beans, dried
- [ ] kidney beans, tin
- [ ] linseed
- [ ] lentils, brown
- [ ] lentils, orange
- [ ] mackerel, tin
- [ ] maple syrup, pure
- [ ] millet meal
- [ ] mountain bread
- [ ] muslin and string for herb bags
- [ ] olive oil, preferably cold pressed
- [ ] oven bags

- [ ] oyster sauce
- [ ] peas, frozen
- [ ] pecan nuts
- [ ] pepita seeds
- [ ] peppercorns, for pepper mill
- [ ] pistachios
- [ ] preserved lemons
- [ ] protein powder
- [ ] prunes, pitted
- [ ] quinoa
- [ ] raisins
- [ ] red curry paste
- [ ] rice crackers, plain
- [ ] rice crackers, seaweed
- [ ] rolled oats
- [ ] salmon, tin
- [ ] sardines, tin
- [ ] sesame seeds
- [ ] spelt flour, white
- [ ] spelt flour, wholemeal
- [ ] spelt pasta, wholemeal
- [ ] stock, chicken
- [ ] stock, beef
- [ ] stock, vegetable

- [ ] sugar, raw
- [ ] sugar, castor
- [ ] sugar, icing
- [ ] sunflower seeds
- [ ] sweet chilli sauce
- [ ] sweet red paprika
- [ ] tahini
- [ ] tamari
- [ ] tea leaves, Earl Grey
- [ ] tea leaves, green
- [ ] tea leaves, lemongrass & ginger
- [ ] tea leaves, liquorice
- [ ] tea leaves, peppermint
- [ ] tuna, tin
- [ ] Thai fish sauce
- [ ] tomatoes diced, tin
- [ ] tomato paste
- [ ] turmeric
- [ ] vanilla beans/vanilla extract
- [ ] walnuts
- [ ] white vinegar
- [ ] wholegrain bread
- [ ] yeast, dried

Fresh food shopping list

MEAT
- [ ] bacon, middle rashers
- [ ] beef, lean minced
- [ ] chicken, breast
- [ ] chicken, whole
- [ ] chicken, thighs
- [ ] fish, fillet
- [ ] lamb, cutlets
- [ ] lamb, steak
- [ ] osso buco
- [ ] steak, rump
- [ ] steak, salmon
- [ ] steak, scotch
- [ ] smoked salmon

SUNDRY
- [ ] sushi
- [ ] miso soup
- [ ] California roll

DAIRY
- [ ] chocolate soy ice-cream
- [ ] eggs

- [ ] feta
- [ ] goat's feta
- [ ] milk
- [ ] mozzarella cheese
- [ ] parmesan cheese
- [ ] ricotta, fresh
- [ ] tofu
- [ ] yoghurt, natural

FRUIT AND VEGETABLES
- [ ] avocado
- [ ] apricots
- [ ] beetroot
- [ ] bok choy
- [ ] broccoli
- [ ] basil
- [ ] blueberries
- [ ] capsicum, red and green
- [ ] carrot
- [ ] celery
- [ ] cherries
- [ ] chillies, red and green
- [ ] coriander

- [ ] cucumber
- [ ] Chinese broccoli
- [ ] Chinese cabbage
- [ ] eggplant
- [ ] garlic
- [ ] ginger
- [ ] green apple
- [ ] green beans
- [ ] grapes
- [ ] kiwifruit
- [ ] leek
- [ ] lemongrass stalk
- [ ] lemons
- [ ] lettuce, cos
- [ ] lettuce, iceberg
- [ ] limes
- [ ] mandarins
- [ ] mint
- [ ] mint, Vietnamese
- [ ] mushrooms, small
- [ ] mushrooms, large
- [ ] nectarines
- [ ] oranges
- [ ] parsley, flat-leaf

- [ ] pineapple
- [ ] pumpkin
- [ ] potato
- [ ] passionfruit
- [ ] peaches
- [ ] parsnip
- [ ] pears
- [ ] rhubarb
- [ ] raspberries
- [ ] radish
- [ ] red cabbage
- [ ] rosemary
- [ ] rocket leaves
- [ ] spanish onions
- [ ] salad leaves
- [ ] strawberries
- [ ] sweet potato
- [ ] spinach leaves
- [ ] spring onions
- [ ] sugar snap peas
- [ ] tomatoes
- [ ] tomatoes, cherry
- [ ] watercress
- [ ] zucchini

Weekly Meal Planner

Date: Sunday 14th March to Saturday 20th March

Each Day choose:
1. A morning juice
2. A breakfast
3. Mid-morning fruit
4. A midday meal
5. An afternoon snack
6. An evening meal

JUICE	BREAKFAST	MID-MORNING FRUIT	MIDDAY MEAL	AFTERNOON SNACK	EVENING MEAL
Pineapple, celery, apple	Baked eggs and spinach with wholegrain toast	2 peaches	Mountain bread wrap of chicken, eggplant dip and salad	Snack pack of nuts, 1 fig	Stir-fried beef and vegetables, piece of chocolate
Apple, celery, carrot, ginger	Bircher muesli with mixed berries	2 slices pineapple	Salmon and salad sandwich on wholegrain bread	Seaweed crackers and eggplant dip	Lamb cutlets with ratatouille and salad, chocolate soy ice-cream with nuts
Beetroot, carrot, celery, ginger, apple	Wholegrain toast with avocado, lemon juice and cracked pepper	1 nectarine, 1 peach	Pea and spinach frittata with ratatouille salad	Vegetable slices with eggplant dip	Lean steak and mixed bean salad, piece of chocolate
Celery, apple, carrot, ginger	Bircher muesli with mixed berries	2 slices pineapple	Nutty quinoa salad	California roll, barley green drink	Herb encrusted salmon and steamed green vegetables, liquorice
Pineapple, celery, apple	Wholegrain toast with tahini and honey	10 fresh cherries	Nicoise salad	Sushi and green barley drink	Lemon roast chicken, pumpkin and green vegetables, piece of chocolate
Apple, celery, carrot, ginger	Bircher muesli with mixed berries	2 slices pineapple	Mountain bread wrap of lemon chicken, goats' feta, eggplant dip, cucumber and rocket leaves	Snack pack of nuts, 1 fig	Spicy bean casserole with salad, chocolate soy ice-cream with nuts
Beetroot, apple, celery, ginger	French toast with tomato and olive salsa	10 fresh cherries	Thai beef salad	Baked ricotta cheese cake	Curried chicken with warm lentil salad

Chapter 16

Kitchen helpers

A healthy kitchen is a kitchen filled with fresh produce. Fresh food markets will supply most of the food you require from your weekly meal planner. Allow a couple of hours of preparation time on shopping day and use a shopping list. Unpack your shopping, portion control as you pack away the food and do some preparation for the coming week.

Preparation ideas

Following are some suggestions for pre-preparation.
- make a dip to use in sandwiches or for an afternoon snack
- make a batch of muesli
- bake a healthy loaf of bread
- roast some pumpkin or sweet potato to add to meals
- marinate meats
- mix up a salad dressing
- bake or poach some fruit
- make a soup, frittata or casserole
- prepare portion-size bags of vegetables to add to an evening meal
- bake a treat like a flourless orange cake or muesli slice
- prepare snack parcels to take to work.

Some of the cakes you bake can be cut into portion-controlled pieces and frozen for ease in future weeks. Muesli can be made in large batches every few weeks and casseroles can be made in larger batches and frozen. Make a little more of some meals and eat them for lunch the next day. When baking a chicken, use your oven and roast some red capsicums, beetroot or eggplant for dips and bake pumpkin pieces to add to meals.

Kitchen Equipment

These items will make preparing meals easier.

Lemon squeezer, blender, grill plate, food processor, juicer, ginger grater, steamer, skillet with ovenproof handle and a teapot.

A variety of large plastic containers are great to replace your refrigerator trays because they keep your vegetables fresh and are really convenient to pull in and out of the refrigerator.

The importance of variety and natural flavours

There is so much information and marketing hype on what individual foods to eat that it can become overwhelming. I always like to be guided by nature and not advertising.

When you look at natural foods there is a lot of variety and different colors. That is a good clue to follow. When it comes to fruits and vegetables, eat lots of different colors. This simple strategy is likely to cover your body's need for many vitamins and trace minerals.

The six tastes of Ayurveda

Ayurvedic medicine identifies that the tongue has six taste receptors. Taste triggers a trail of reactions from your mouth to the food's final destination, your cells. The six tastes are salty, sweet, sour, bitter, astringent and pungent. Food falls into these six categories in the following ways:
- Fruits – primarily sweet and astringent, with citrus fruits adding sour.
- Vegetables – primarily sweet and astringent, with leafy greens adding bitter.
- Dairy – primarily sweet, with yoghurt and cheese adding sour and astringent.
- Meat – primarily sweet and astringent.
- Oils – primarily sweet.
- Grains and nuts – primarily sweet and astringent.
- Legumes – primarily sweet and astringent.
- Herbs and spices – primarily pungent, with all other tastes secondary.
- Celtic, sea and vegetable salts – salty.

Variety is the spice of life

Set up your kitchen with a variety of foods, herbs and spices that give delicious flavour to your meals. If you add interesting flavours, you will wake up your taste buds and feel more satisfied.

Eat a wide variety of natural foods to satisfy all the tastes on your tongue and add spices and natural flavours to your meals. Stock up with the following:

DRIED HERBS
Sweet red paprika, cumin, coriander, garam masala, coriander, turmeric, chilli and Celtic sea salt.

FAVORITE SPICE MIX
Mix together the following spices and place in an airtight jar. Use the mix to flavour soups and stews.
  4 tablespoons dried coriander
  4 tablespoons ground cumin
  2 tablespoons garam masala
  2 tablespoons sweet red paprika

FRESH HERBS
Flat-leaf parsley, mint, coriander, dill, basil, curry leaves, rosemary, chives, oregano, marjoram, thyme, sage, garlic, lemongrass, ginger, red and green chilli.

ROSEMARY FLAVOUR BAG

Rosemary is easy to grow in your garden or in a pot. It adds a rich flavour to stews and soups. Cut out squares of muslin and fill with rosemary stems then tie with string. These flavour pouches can then be placed in your cooking pots and removed at the end of the cooking.

FLAVOUR ENHANCERS

Low-salt stock, dry white wine, cold pressed olive oil, low-salt tamari, the fresh juice of oranges, lemons, limes, and mandarins, Dijon mustard, red and green curry paste.

MARINADES

When you unpack your shopping, place your meats in your chosen marinade and store in your fridge or freezer. They will be deliciously marinated when you are ready to cook them.

Some marinade suggestions include:
- natural yoghurt, curry paste, lime juice and mint
- dry white wine, garlic and olive oil
- olive oil, favorite spice mix and fresh rosemary
- freshly squeezed orange juice, tamari, freshly grated ginger, dry white wine

Opposite page:
Rosemary flavour bag

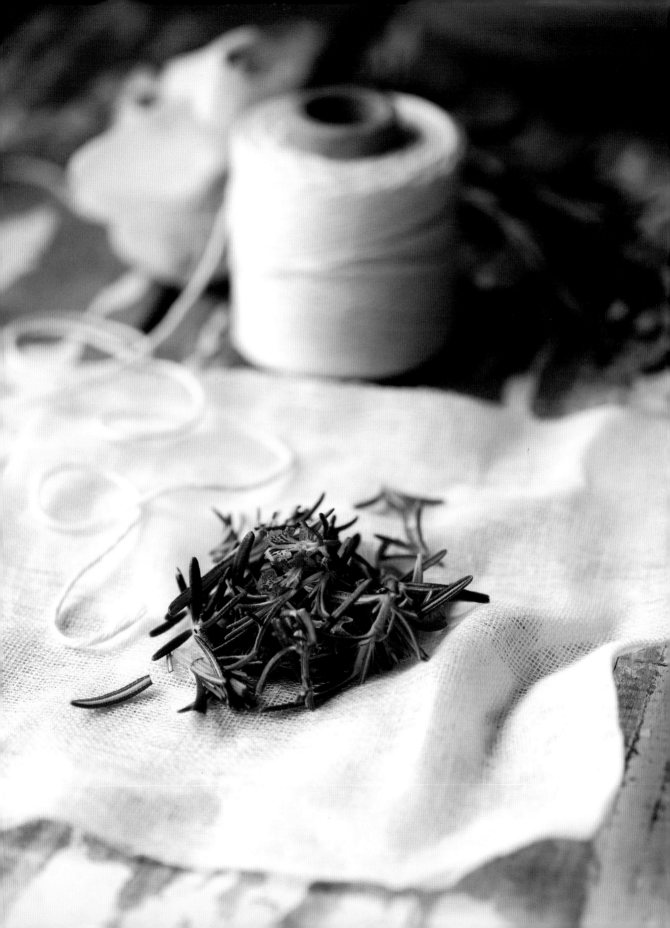

HANDY DIPS

Another helpful strategy is to make flavourful dips that can be added to your meals. If you do this at the beginning of the week you will be well prepared to easily add flavour to your meals. Dips served with raw vegetable sticks or rice crackers are a nourishing afternoon snack or great just before dinner when you are on the hunt for a quick snack. If you have prepared healthy dips, it's less likely that you and your family will snack on unhealthy food.

Hummus

> 1 x 400–425g (14.5–15 oz) can chickpeas
> 2 tablespoons tahini
> juice of two large lemons
> 1/4 teaspoon cumin or favorite spice mix
>   (see p95)
> 1/4 teaspoon Celtic salt
> 1 small garlic clove, crushed

Blend all ingredients in a food processor until smooth. If the mixture is dry add water or olive oil one teaspoon at a time until the right consistency is achieved.

Eggplant dip

> 1 large eggplant
> 1 small garlic clove, crushed
> juice of 1 lemon
> 1 tablespoon tahini
> 2 tablespoons natural yoghurt
> 1/4 teaspoon ground cumin or favorite
>   spice mix (see p95)
> pinch of Celtic sea salt

Preheat oven to 180°C (350°F).

Prick the eggplant with a skewer and place on a tray in the oven. The eggplant is cooked when it is soft to the touch.

Remove the eggplant from the oven, place in a bowl and cover with plastic. Set aside to cool.

Halve the eggplant and scoop out the flesh. Place in a food processor with remaining ingredients and blend until smooth.

Minted yoghurt dip

> 1 cup natural yoghurt
> handful of fresh mint, finely chopped
> 8 cm (3 in) length cucumber, grated

Gently combine all ingredients and place in an airtight container.

Coriander can be used in place of the mint.

Pesto

Pesto is so versatile. It's a great base for things on toast. It's delicious on top of vegetable soup or spread on sandwiches. It's also good topped on meat or fish and is a delicious filler for stuffed vegetables.

Homemade pesto is full of enzymes and antioxidants, protein, calcium, essential fatty acids and fibre, and is a great lubricant for your digestive system.

> 1/4 cup almonds or walnuts
> pinch of Celtic sea salt
> 1 bunch basil, leaves only
> 5 tablespoons olive oil
> 1/4 cup parmesan cheese, finely grated

Place nuts and salt in a food processor and blend to a smooth paste.

Add the basil leaves and a drizzle of olive oil. Process until the leaves are chopped. Gradually add more olive oil while the processor is running until the mixture is smooth. Stir in parmesan cheese. If the mixture is dry add a little more olive oil.

Crushed garlic or 1/4 cup of pitted black olives can be added for extra flavour. Flat-leaf parsley, coriander or rocket can be used instead of basil to make pesto.

Opposite page:
A selection of kitchen helpers

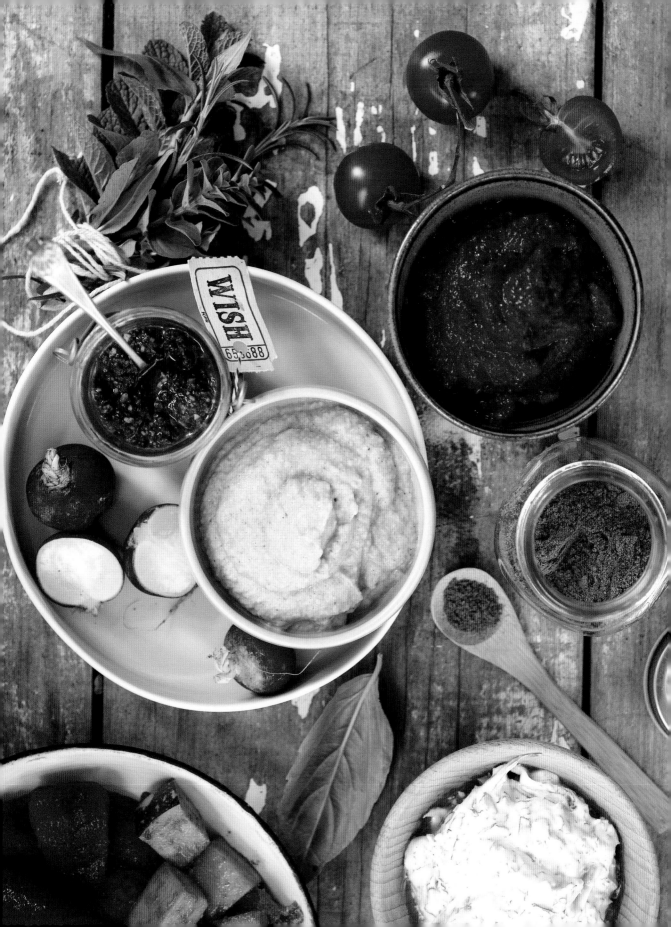

Beetroot dip

Beetroot has a high sodium and potassium content which gives it blood-cleansing abilities. Natural sodium expels toxins and helps maintain normal blood pressure. Other benefits include aiding digestion and cleansing the lymphatic system and the kidneys.

> 1 large beetroot, scrubbed and trimmed
> juice of half lemon
> pinch Celtic sea salt
> 1 small clove garlic, crushed
> ¼ teaspoon favorite spice mix (see p95)
> ¼ cup natural yoghurt

Preheat oven to 180°C (350°F).

Place beetroot on a tray covered with baking paper and place in oven. Cook for about one hour or until a skewer can be inserted easily into the beetroot. Set aside to cool slightly.

When cool enough to handle, peel off outside skin and roughly chop beetroot. Place in a food processor with lemon juice, garlic, Celtic sea salt and favorite spice mix. Blend until smooth. Add the yoghurt and stir to combine.

ROASTED VEGETABLES

Roasted red capsicums

> 4 red capsicums

Preheat oven to 180°C (350°F).

Place whole capsicums on an oven tray and bake for 1 hour.

Remove capsicums from oven, place in a bowl and cover with plastic. Set aside to cool.

When cool, you will easily be able to peel off the skins and discard the seeds. Cut into pieces and store in an airtight container in the fridge.

Add to salads, sandwiches and wraps.

Roasted pumpkin pieces

> ¼ Jap pumpkin, peeled and cut into 3 cm (1 in) pieces
> 1 tablespoon olive oil
> ½ teaspoon favorite spice mix (see p95)

Preheat oven to 180°C (350°F).

Place ingredients in a plastic bag and seal. Shake to coat the pumpkin with the oil and spice mix.

Tip out onto an oven tray lined with baking paper. Bake until soft and golden brown in color.

When cooled the pumpkin can be stored in the fridge and used in salads and sandwiches or reheated to add to a meal. Sweet potato can also be used instead of pumpkin.

VEGETABLE PARCELS

Another handy way to prepare vegetables to save time on those busy days is to prepare a variety of vegetables in portion servings before you pack them in the fridge. Try green beans, broccoli, cauliflower, sugar snap peas, zucchini or bok choy.

Cut the vegetables into bite-sized pieces and put them in a sealable bag or container. They are then easy to steam and serve with fish, lamb, chicken or beef that has been marinated.

When serving steamed vegetables, squeeze fresh orange or mandarin juice over the top and sprinkle with chopped walnuts.

Opposite page:
Preparing pumpkin for roasting

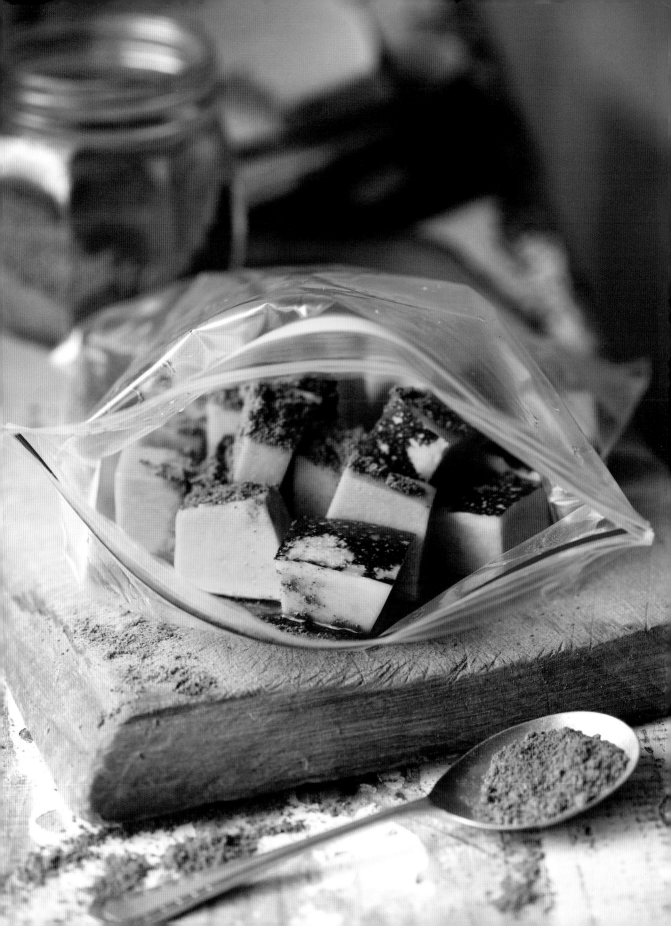

NOURISHING BREAD

Breads vary greatly in quality, nutritional value and flavour. Choose wholegrain breads because they are low GI.

Making your own bread allows you to choose and have control over the ingredients. I recommend using spelt flour rather than wheat flour. Spelt provides more of the essential elements needed by the body. It's higher in protein than wheat flour and has B17, which has anti-cancer properties.

Millet is another grain that also contains B17. Before modernisation of our food chain most bread was made from millet meal. You can add a small amount of ground millet to enrich the bread you make.

Machine-made spelt bread

- 2 cups wholemeal spelt flour
- 1 cup spelt white flour
- 1 cup lukewarm water, plus an extra splash
- $\frac{1}{2}$ teaspoon Celtic sea salt
- 1 teaspoon sugar
- 2 teaspoons dried yeast
- 1 tablespoon oil
- $\frac{1}{4}$ cup linseeds
- 2 tablespoons millet meal

Place all ingredients in the breadmaker and follow your breadmaker instructions.

Hand-made spelt bread

Use the same ingredients as machine-made spelt bread and combine in a large mixing bowl to form a soft dough.

Lightly flour your work surface and knead the dough for about 5 minutes or until smooth and elastic.

Place the dough back in the bowl and cover with a clean tea towel dampened with hot water.

Place in a warm draught-free spot until the bread dough doubles in size. This is called proving the dough and will take about $1\frac{1}{4}$ to 2 hours.

Punch the dough down to remove the air and turn out onto the floured work surface. Knead again for about 5 minutes. Shape the dough into a loaf.

Place the dough in a floured bread tin, cover again with the dampened tea towel and set aside to prove for another hour or until the dough doubles in size.

Preheat your oven to 200°C (400°F).

Bake for about 30 minutes or until golden brown. Your sense of smell will tell you that your homemade bread is ready. You can also tap the bottom of the bread and if it sounds hollow, it is cooked.

The Metabolic Clock Recipes

The following recipes are everyday meals designed for busy people who want to enjoy food in its most natural and nourishing way. When creating your weekly meal plan make one selection from each of the following sections for each day of the week. If you have any food allergies, just make adjustments to the ingredients.

Note: each recipe specifies the number of meals it makes. Each recipe can easily be doubled or multiplied depending on the number of meals required. Some recipes allow for leftovers or for portions to be frozen for another meal.

MORNING JUICE

You have been fasting throughout the night so your body needs rehydrating and detoxifying. A great way to do this is with a freshly prepared morning juice. A fresh juice will fill your body with life-giving enzymes and the antioxidants will flush away toxins accumulated from the healing processes that took place during sleep. Your digestive system does not have to work hard to process the juice and you'll be giving your body a morning dose of vitamins and minerals that will increase energy and improve mental alertness.

Invest in a good juicing machine to make your morning elixir. If you don't have a juicer, start your day with hot water and the juice of half a lemon. You can add 1 teaspoon of honey as a sweetener if you prefer.

Celery is a good base for juices. It's a weight watcher's dream food because it's low in calories and high in minerals. Celery juice reduces arthritic inflammation, is a diuretic, replaces lost sodium salts and stimulates the pancreas to assist in carbohydrate digestion. Here are some delicious juice combinations.

- carrot, celery and a slice of ginger
- carrot, celery and green apple
- celery, green apple and pineapple
- celery, carrot, small piece of beetroot, sprig of parsley
- cucumber, mint leaves, celery, green apple
- grapes, celery and green apple
- strawberries, green apple and celery
- green apple, celery, ginger, beetroot

You can experiment with any combination of fruits and vegetables, except for oranges: they are best juiced on their own.

Opposite page:
A selection of juices

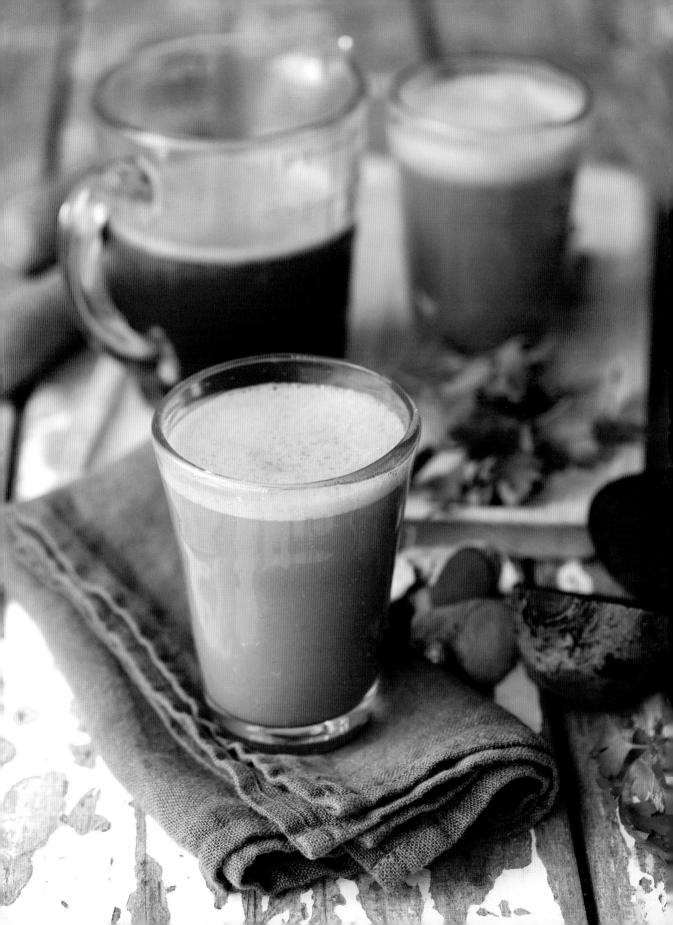

BREAKFAST

Eating breakfast is very important. It's the meal that breaks the fasting and healing process that has taken place during the night. It's also essential to kick-start your metabolism and provide fuel for the day's activities. Make breakfast an important meal in your wellness strategy. When making your weekly meal plan choose from the following breakfast ideas.

- muesli (see p108)with poached pears and yoghurt
- porridge
- Bircher muesli
- hard-boiled eggs with wholegrain toast
- tomato and olive open-faced omelette
- poached eggs (tomatoes and mushrooms can be added)
- poached eggs with spinach and salmon slices
- sautéed mushrooms with wilted spinach and goat's feta
- french toast with fresh herb, tomato and olive salsa
- home-made baked beans on wholegrain bread
- toppings for toast
- baked rhubarb and apples with yoghurt and muesli
- baked apples with dates, nuts and yoghurt

Muesli with poached pears and yoghurt

2 meals

1 cup apple juice
1 cup water
1 tablespoon of currants
half a fresh vanilla bean or ½ teaspoon vanilla extract
2 firm pears, peeled
½ cup homemade muesli base
¼ cup natural yoghurt

Place a small saucepan over medium heat. Add apple juice, water, currants and vanilla and bring to the boil. Reduce heat to low, add pears and simmer for 15 to 20 minutes or until tender. Remove pears with a slotted spoon and set aside. Increase heat and reduce the syrup by half. Core the pears and slice in half.

Serve warm or cooled in a bowl with the syrup, muesli and yoghurt.

Note: Peaches and nectarines can also be poached in this way.

Opposite page: Muesli with poached pears and yoghurt

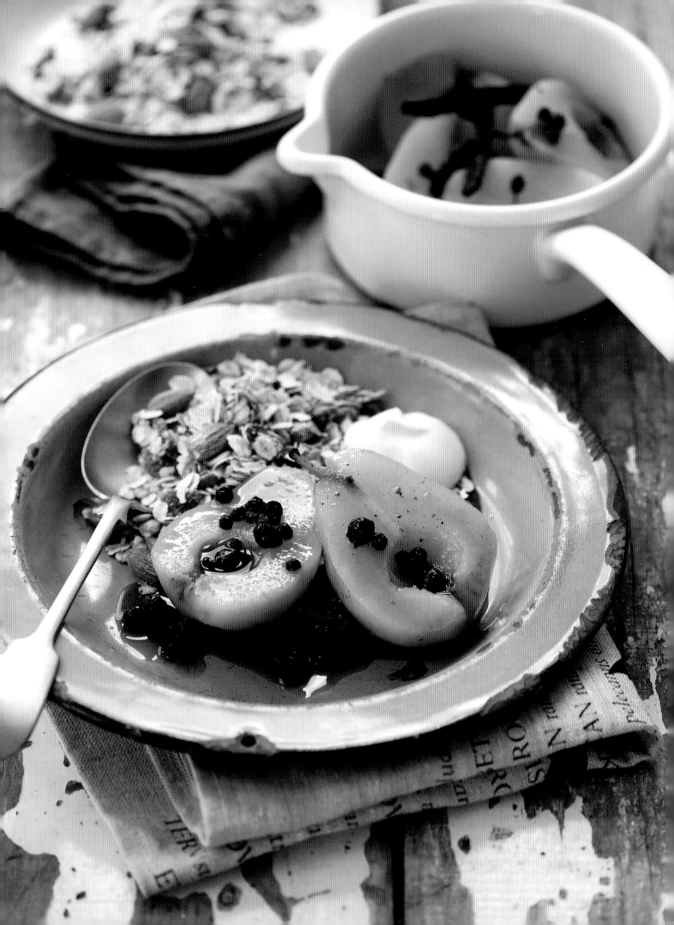

Porridge

1 meal

½ cup rolled oats
1 cup water, for soaking
1½ cups water, extra
pinch of Celtic sea salt

Before going to bed, place rolled oats and soaking water in a small saucepan and leave to soak overnight.

Next morning, drain the water off the oats and add the extra water. Place the saucepan over medium heat, stir frequently with a wooden spoon and bring to the boil. Reduce heat and continue to cook for another 3 to 4 minutes or until oats are soft and creamy.

Stir in salt and serve immediately with your favorite topping.

Toppings for porridge include:

- a splash of milk and a dash of brown sugar or honey
- soy milk or rice milk and honey
- a small handful of almonds and raisins or prunes
- pure maple syrup and milk

Easy muesli base

Homemade muesli is nourishing and makes a very handy breakfast. You can also use it to make yummy slices. It provides protein, essential fatty acids and fibre to give your digestive system a good workout. It also gives you energy from carbohydrates. Oats contain a special ingredient in the fibre called betaglucan. This helps to slow the rise in blood sugar levels and reduce blood cholesterol. You can add extra ingredients to 'customise' your muesli. Try prunes, dates, raisins, dried apricots, sunflower or pepita seeds or pecan nuts.

Makes 5 cups

3 cups rolled oats
¼ cup linseeds
¼ cup sesame seeds
½ cup currants
½ cup of almonds, roughly chopped or left whole
½ cup Brazil nuts, roughly chopped

In a large bowl mix all the ingredients together with a large spoon or with your hands. Place in a large glass jar with a good fitting lid.

Bircher muesli

1 meal

½ cup muesli base
½ cup apple or apple and pear juice
½ cup water
¼ cup natural yoghurt
fresh berries, peach slices, kiwifruit, passionfruit or any seasonal fruit of your choice

Place muesli in a small bowl and add juice and water. Soak overnight.

The next morning stir through yoghurt and top with fresh berries, peach slices, kiwifruit or passionfruit.

Hard-boiled eggs with wholegrain toast

1 meal

2 free-range or organic eggs (at room temperature)
1 slice wholegrain bread

Place a saucepan filled with water over high heat and bring to the boil. Carefully lower the eggs into the water with a spoon. Reduce heat and simmer for 3 minutes.

Remove the eggs and run under cold water to stop them from cooking further. Place in egg cups. Toast the bread and serve with the hard-boiled eggs.

Tomato and olive open-faced omelette

1 meal

1 teaspoon olive oil
3 cm (1 in) length leek, white part only, thinly sliced
2 large free-range or organic eggs
pinch of Celtic sea salt
cracked black pepper
3 black olives, stoned and chopped
4 cherry tomatoes, halved
25 g (1 oz) goat's feta, crumbled
1 slice wholegrain bread
large handful of watercress or rocket leaves, washed and well dried

Place a non-stick, ovenproof frying pan 15 cm (6 in) diameter over a medium heat. Add olive oil and sauté leek for 3 to 5 minutes, stirring occasionally. If making 2 meals double the mixture and use an 20 cm (8 in) frying pan.

Whisk the eggs with the salt and add to the pan.

Sprinkle the olives, cherry tomatoes and goat's feta evenly over top of the egg mixture. Cook on a gentle heat for another 3 minutes while preheating the grill.

Place pan under grill for another 5 minutes or until golden. Toast bread.

Serve the omelette with rocket or watercress leaves, cracked pepper and toast.

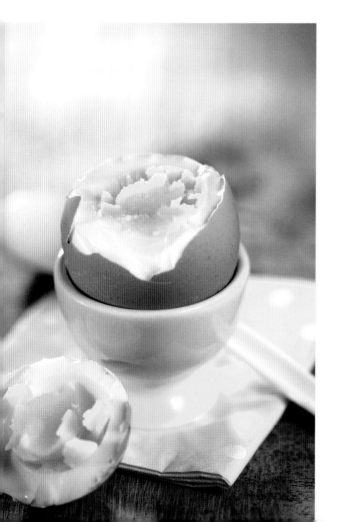

A hard-boiled egg

Poached eggs

1 meal

2 free-range or organic eggs
1 tablespoon white vinegar
pinch of Celtic sea salt
1 slice wholegrain bread
flat-leaf parsley, finely chopped
cracked black pepper

Break each egg into a cup to ensure the yolk is intact.

Fill a deep-sided saucepan with at least 10 cm (4 in) of simmering water. Add the vinegar and a pinch of salt to the water. Stir the water with a spoon, creating a small whirlpool. Drop each egg into the centre of the whirlpool and wait for 3 to 4 minutes. The water will settle and the eggs should form an oval.

While the eggs are cooking toast the bread.

Remove the eggs with a slotted spoon and drain well. Place the eggs on the toast, sprinkle with parsley and cracked black pepper.

Note: You might also like to spread pesto or goat's feta on the toast and add sautéed tomatoes and mushrooms.

Poached eggs with spinach and salmon slices

1 meal

large handful baby spinach leaves, washed
2 free-range or organic eggs
1 tablespoon white vinegar
pinch of Celtic sea salt
1 slice wholegrain bread
lemon half, to squeeze
cracked black pepper
2 slices smoked salmon

Place spinach leaves in a shallow frypan and heat until wilted (about 2 to 3 minutes). The water clinging to the leaves will steam the leaves gently. Remove, drain well and set aside.

Break each egg into a cup to ensure the yolk is intact.

Fill a deep-sided saucepan with at least 10 cm (4 in) of simmering water. Add the vinegar and a pinch of salt to the water. Stir the water with a spoon, creating a small whirlpool. Drop each egg in the centre of the whirlpool and cook for 3 to 4 minutes. The water will settle and the eggs should form an oval.

While the eggs are cooking toast the bread.

Remove the eggs with a slotted spoon, drain well and set aside.

Dress the spinach with a squeeze of lemon juice and season with salt and pepper. Place the spinach on the toast, add the salmon slices followed by the poached eggs. Serve immediately.

Opposite page: Poached eggs with spinach and salmon slices

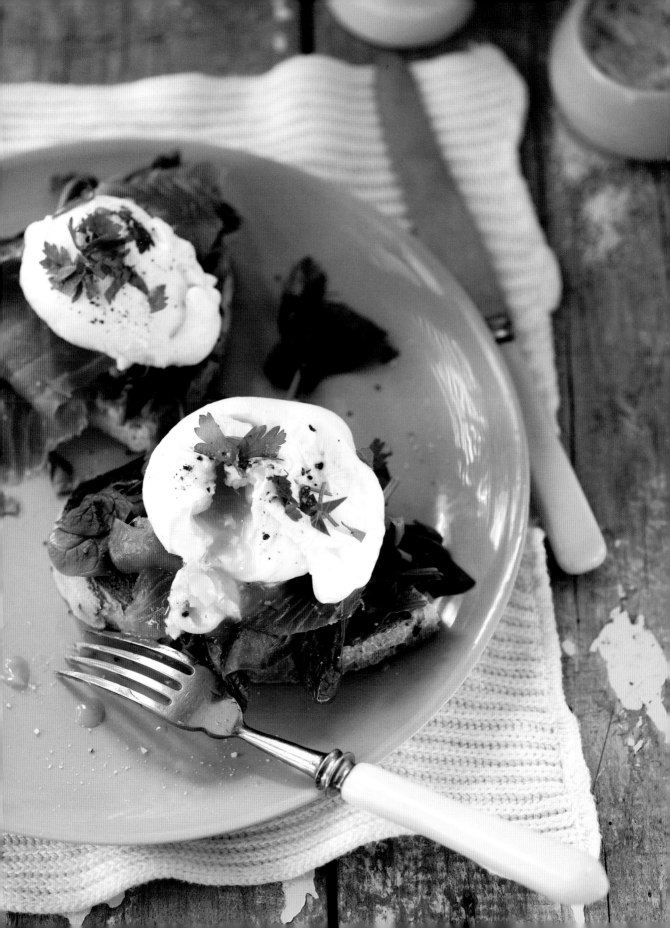

Sautéed mushrooms with wilted spinach and goat's feta

1 meal

1 teaspoon olive oil
2–3 large field mushrooms or 4 Swiss brown mushrooms, halved
pinch of Celtic sea salt and cracked black pepper
large handful baby spinach leaves, washed
1 thick slice wholegrain bread
25 g (1 oz) goat's feta
½ lemon, to squeeze
flat-leaf parsley, finely chopped

Place a non-stick frying pan over medium heat. Add olive oil and heat.

Add the mushrooms to the pan with salt and cracked pepper. Place a lid on the pan and cook until mushrooms are tender, turning them occasionally during cooking. Add water if the mixture looks dry.

When mushrooms are cooked, add spinach and replace lid. Cook for 3 minutes.

Toast the bread and spread evenly with goat's feta. Place on serving plate. Pile mushrooms and spinach on toast, squeeze over lemon and sprinkle with parsley.

French toast with herb, tomato and olive salsa

1 meal

2 free-range or organic eggs
splash milk
pinch of Celtic sea salt and cracked black pepper
1 teaspoon olive oil
6 cherry tomatoes, finely diced
6 pitted black olives, finely diced
1 spring onion or ¼ Spanish onion, finely diced
6 basil leaves or a handful of coriander leaves, roughly torn
25 g (1 oz) goat's feta or feta
1 slice crusty wholegrain bread
large handful rocket leaves, washed and well dried

In a small, flat bowl whisk eggs, milk, salt and cracked pepper. Place a non-stick frying pan over medium heat and add olive oil to heat.

For the salsa, combine the tomatoes, olives, onion, basil leaves and feta or goat's feta in a small bowl.

Dip the bread in egg mixture until well covered. Add to pan and cook on both sides until golden brown and slightly crisp. Place on serving plate, top with salsa mixture and rocket.

Note: If the ingredients for the salsa are not available you can use bottled gourmet chutney.

Opposite page: French toast with herb, tomato and olive salsa

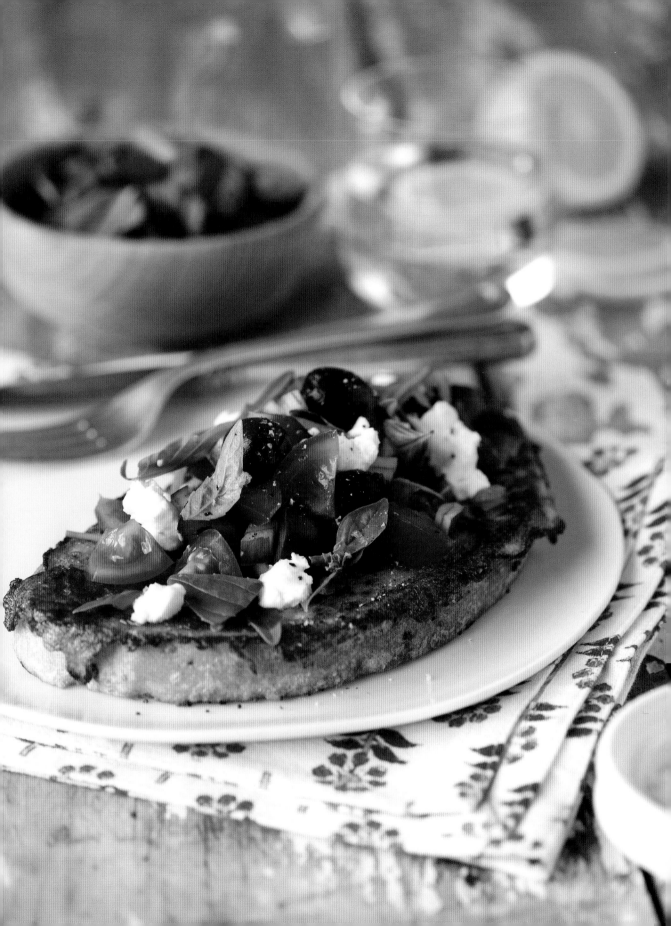

Homemade baked beans on wholegrain toast

4 meals

1 teaspoon olive oil

1 small onion, finely chopped

1 clove garlic, crushed

2 pieces middle rasher bacon, finely diced

¼ cup dry white wine

4 cups hot water

1 cup dried cannellini beans (soaked overnight in water, well drained)

50 g (1.75 oz) sweet potato, peeled and diced

2 teaspoons tomato paste

1 cup of vegetable or beef stock

1 rosemary flavour bag (see p96)

1 teaspoon favorite spice mix (see p95)

2 tablespoons flat-leaf parsley, finely chopped

fresh or dried chilli, to taste

1 slice crusty wholegrain bread

Place a large heavy-based saucepan over medium heat and add olive oil. Add onion, garlic and bacon and sauté for 3 minutes, then add the wine and hot water. Bring to the boil and add beans and remaining ingredients. Reduce heat and simmer for an hour or until the beans are tender. Serve on wholegrain toast and sprinkle with parsley.

Note: As an option a handful of spinach leaves can be stirred into the cooked beans just before serving.

Toppings for toast

Always use multigrain or spelt bread for a lower GI effect. Use these combinations to add a bit of variety to your morning toast.

- goat's feta and pesto topped with slices of fresh tomato
- mashed avocado seasoned with lemon juice and cracked black pepper
- smoked salmon and mashed avocado
- ricotta cheese with a pure fruit spread
- tahini with honey

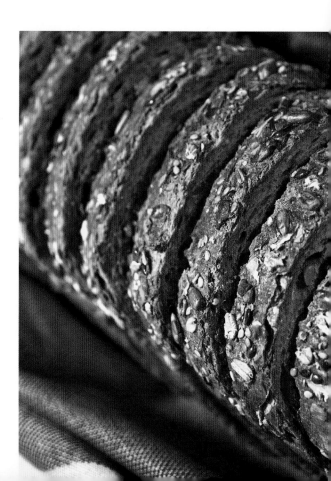

For a lower GI effect, always use multigrain or spelt bread for your toast

114

Baked rhubarb and apple with yoghurt and muesli

1 meal and enough fruit for 4 meals

2 Granny Smith apples, peeled, cored and thinly sliced
300 g (10.5 oz) rhubarb, cut into 4 cm (1.5 in) lengths
2 tablespoons raw sugar
¼ cup organic apple juice
¼ cup of muesli
½ cup natural yoghurt

Preheat oven to 180°C (350°F).

Place fruit in baking dish and sprinkle with raw sugar and apple juice. Cover with aluminium foil and bake for 40 minutes. Cool with the foil on.

Serve warm or cold with natural yoghurt and muesli.

Note: Meal portions of the fruit can be frozen and eaten later.

Baked apples with dates, nuts and yoghurt

2 meals

8 walnuts, roughly chopped
4 dates, roughly chopped
1 tablespoon raw sugar
2 Granny Smith apples, cored
½ cup organic apple juice
½ cup natural yoghurt

Preheat the oven to 180°C (350°F).

In a small bowl mix the walnuts, dates and sugar together.

Score the apples around the middle horizontally, just cutting through the skins and place in a baking dish. Pour over apple juice. Fill the apples with the nut mixture and cover with aluminium foil.

Bake for 20 minutes or until the apples are tender, but still holding their shape.

Serve warm or cold with natural yoghurt.

Note: You can add ¼ cup of muesli or ground almonds to add variety to this breakfast.

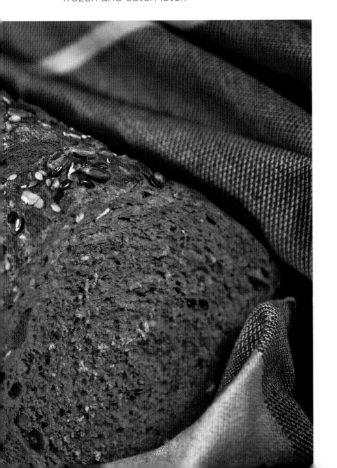

MID-MORNING FRUIT

Eating raw fruit mid-morning will provide you with life-giving enzymes that will speed up your metabolism. The fibre and water content in the fruit will create the right variables for digestive vitality. Make sure you include lots of variety for the antioxidants and trace minerals.

If you are hungry after eating mid-morning fruit this means that your metabolism is speeding up and you can look forward to enjoying your midday meal.

Choose one of the following for your mid-morning fruit.

- 2 slices of pineapple
- 5 cherries and a peach
- 1 pear and 1 kiwifruit
- 2 kiwifruit
- 1 peach and 1 passionfruit
- 1 pear and 1 apple
- 2 mandarins
- small bunch grapes
- 2 apricots
- 1 nectarine and a peach
- 1 peach and 6 raspberries
- 1 slice rockmelon or honeydew melon and 4 strawberries
- 4 strawberries, 8 blueberries and 8 raspberries

Opposite page:
A selection of fresh fruit

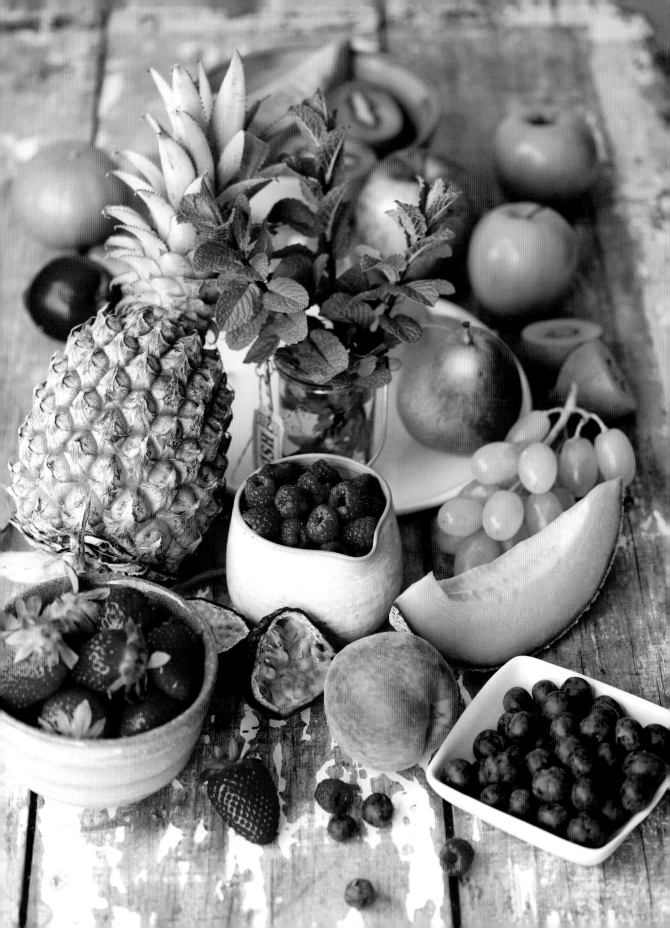

MIDDAY MEAL

Eat a sustaining meal close to midday. At this time of day your metabolism is most efficient for digesting food. Add carbohydrates and protein to this meal to create the energy for your afternoon activities. When making your weekly meal plan choose from the following midday meals:

- vegetable and bean soup with pesto
- chicken soup with wholegrain bread
- mountain bread wraps with fillings
- pesto field mushrooms
- dhal with kidney beans
- sardines or mackerel on wholegrain bread
- meal salad
- quinoa and chicken salad
- nutty quinoa salad
- chicken sandwich
- tuna or salmon sandwich
- pea and spinach frittata with salad
- wholemeal or spelt pasta with fresh tomato and basil sauce
- Thai beef salad
- Niçoise salad
- try the egg recipes or homemade baked beans from the breakfast menu on p106

Opposite page: Vegetable and bean soup with pesto

Vegetable and bean soup with pesto

This soup is comforting to have as your midday or evening meal. You can try different vegetables to vary the flavour.

4 meals

1 teaspoon olive oil
1 large onion, finely diced
2 garlic cloves, crushed
2 celery stalks, diced
1 x 400–425g (14.5–15 oz) can diced Roma tomatoes
1 tablespoon tomato paste
1 large carrot, diced
1 small sweet potato, diced
1 teaspoon favorite spice mix (see p95)
1 rosemary flavour bag (see p96)
6 cups hot water
1½ cups vegetable stock or beef stock
1 cup dried borlotti beans (soaked overnight in water, well drained)
1 small potato, grated
1 cup green beans, sliced
1 teaspoon homemade pesto, per meal (see p98)
4 slices wholegrain bread, to serve

Place a large heavy-based saucepan with a tight fitting lid over medium heat. Add olive oil and sauté onion, garlic and celery for 3 minutes.

Add canned tomatoes, tomato paste, carrots, sweet potato, favorite spice mix, rosemary herb bag, hot water, stock, borlotti beans and grated potato. The starch in the potato will thicken the soup slightly. Bring to boil, then reduce heat and simmer uncovered for about one and a half hours until beans are tender. Remove from heat, remove the rosemary flavour bag and stir through green beans.

Ladle soup into a serving bowl and top each meal serve with a teaspoon of pesto. Serve with wholegrain bread per meal.

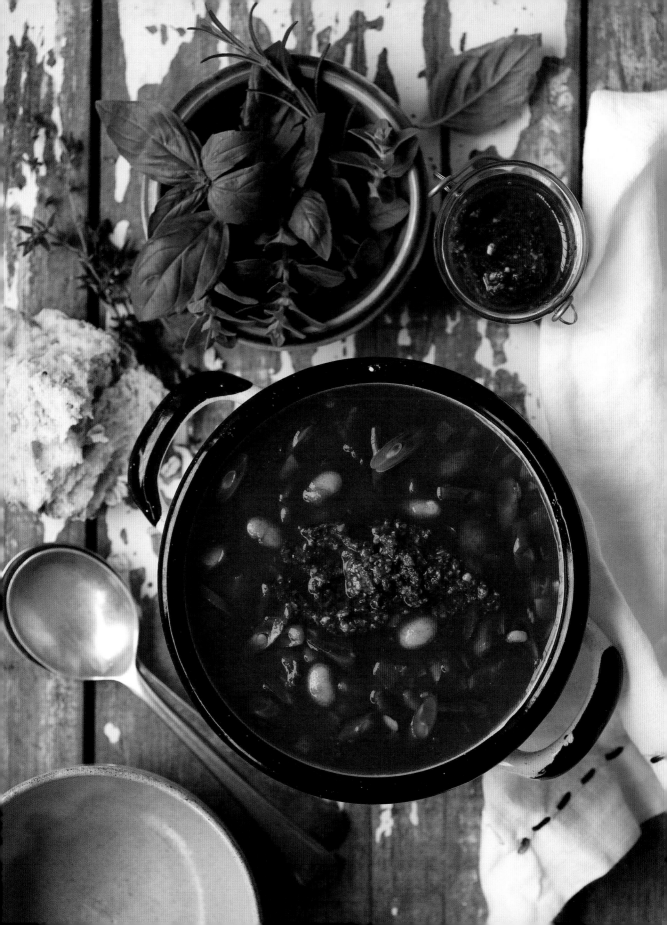

Chicken soup with wholegrain bread

4 meals

1 teaspoon olive oil
10 cm (4 in) piece leek, white part only, finely chopped
2 garlic cloves, crushed
1 carrot, peeled and diced
1 parsnip, diced
1 celery stalk, diced
2 chicken thighs
6 cups hot water
1½ cups chicken stock
½ teaspoon cumin
½ cup pearl barley
¼ cup flat-leaf parsley, finely chopped
wholegrain bread, to serve

Place a large heavy-based saucepan with a tight fitting lid over medium heat. Add oil and sauté leek, garlic, carrot, parsnip and celery for 3 minutes.

Add chicken thighs, hot water, stock and cumin. Cover and simmer for 40 minutes.

Remove the chicken and cool. When cool enough to handle, remove skin and finely shred chicken meat. Set aside.

Add the pearl barley to the soup mix and cook for 30 minutes. Return chicken meat to soup and warm the chicken through. Ladle into soup bowls and sprinkle with parsley. Serve with wholegrain bread.

Opposite page: A hummus, cucumber, roasted pumpkin, tomato and rocket wrap

Mountain bread wraps

Try filling mountain bread wraps with:

- cooked chicken or canned salmon with salad
- mashed avocado, pesto and salad
- cooked and mashed pumpkin, goat's feta and salad
- goat's feta, roasted capsicum, eggplant dip and baby spinach
- hummus, cucumber, roasted pumpkin, tomato and rocket
- pear slices, avocado, cucumber and rocket
- lemon chicken, minted yoghurt, cucumber, Spanish onion and baby spinach

Pesto field mushrooms

1 meal

2 thick slices wholegrain bread, stale is best
¼ cup pesto (see p98)
2 tablespoons pistachios
pinch of Celtic sea salt and cracked pepper
¼ cup parmesan cheese, finely grated
2 large field mushrooms, wiped and stalks removed
salad or steamed green vegetables, to serve

Preheat oven to 180°C (350°F).

Place stale bread in food processor and process to fine crumbs. In a small bowl, combine pesto with breadcrumbs, pistachios, salt, pepper and parmesan cheese.

Place mushrooms, cap side down on a lined baking tray. Fill the cups with pesto mixture and bake for 20 minutes.

Serve with a salad of your choice or steamed green vegetables.

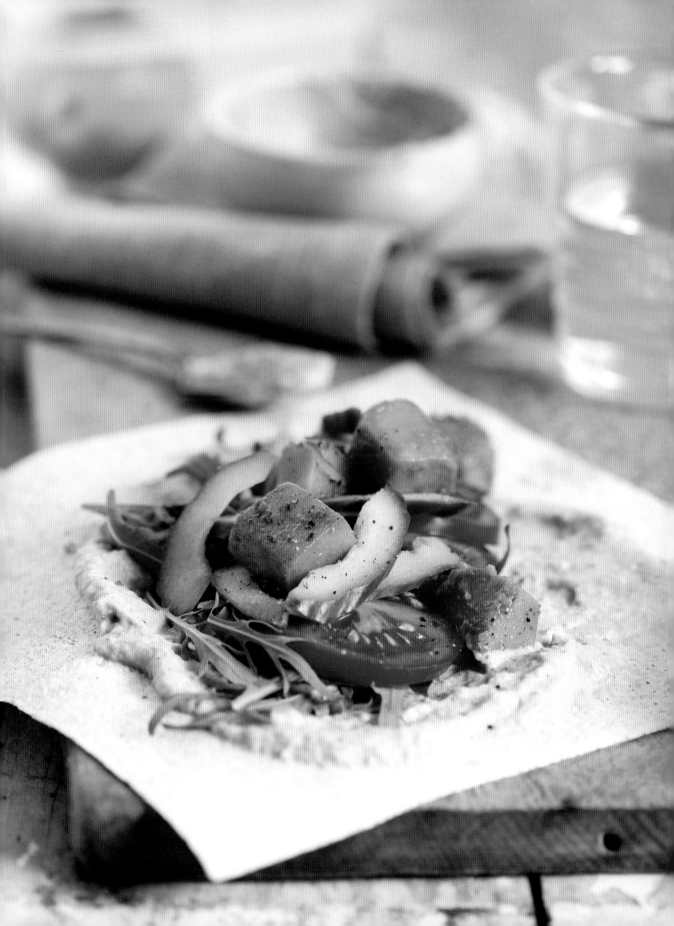

Dhal with kidney beans

4 meals

5 cups water

pinch of Celtic sea salt

1 cup red lentils, rinsed and picked over
   to remove dirt

1 teaspoon olive oil

1 onion, finely diced

2 cloves garlic, crushed

8 cm (3 in) piece sweet potato, finely diced

½ teaspoon turmeric

1 tablespoon grated ginger

1 teaspoon red curry paste

1 teaspoon favorite spice mix (see p95)

½ cup dry white wine

1 cup chicken or vegetable stock

1 tablespoon tomato paste

1 x 400–425g (14.5–15 oz) can kidney
   beans, rinsed and drained

¼ cup natural yoghurt

6 cm (2.5 in) piece cucumber, grated and
   well drained

1 chapatti

coriander, finely chopped

Place a large heavy based saucepan over
medium high heat. Add water and pinch of
salt and bring to a simmer. Add lentils to the
simmering water and cook until lentils are
cooked but not soft. Drain well.

Place a large saucepan over medium heat,
add olive oil, onion, garlic, sweet potato
and turmeric and sauté for 3 minutes. Add
grated ginger, red curry paste, spice mix,
white wine, stock, tomato paste, drained
lentils and kidney beans.

Cook for 10 minutes, stirring occasionally,
adding water if the mixture becomes dry.

In a small bowl combine natural yoghurt and
cucumber and set aside.

Place a non-stick frying pan over high heat
and dry-fry chapatti on both sides.

To serve, spoon dhal into bowls, top with
yoghurt with cucumber. Sprinkle with
coriander and serve with chapatti bread.

Sardines (or mackerel) on wholegrain bread

This is a simple and quick meal that will
satisfy. It's full of essential fatty acids and
protein. You can also toast the bread if
you prefer.

1 meal

1 x 110 g (3.75 oz) can of sardines or
   mackerel, drained and mashed

2 slices wholegrain bread

½ lemon, to squeeze

pinch of Celtic sea salt and cracked
   pepper

Spread the sardines or mackerel evenly over
bread slices, then add a squeeze of lemon
juice. Season with salt and cracked pepper.

Meal salad

Prepare a large salad of your favorite fresh
ingredients such as different varieties of
lettuce, baby spinach, mint, coriander,
watercress, cucumber, celery, cherry
tomatoes, carrots, avocado, Spanish onion,
sprouts, flat-leaf parsley, red and green
capsicum, currants, walnuts, feta or goat's
feta. Add cooked chicken, salmon or tuna,
poached eggs, a piece of lean, red meat,
or cooked lima beans. Drizzle with your
favorite salad dressing and enjoy this simple
and sustaining meal.

Opposite page:
A selection of salad leaves

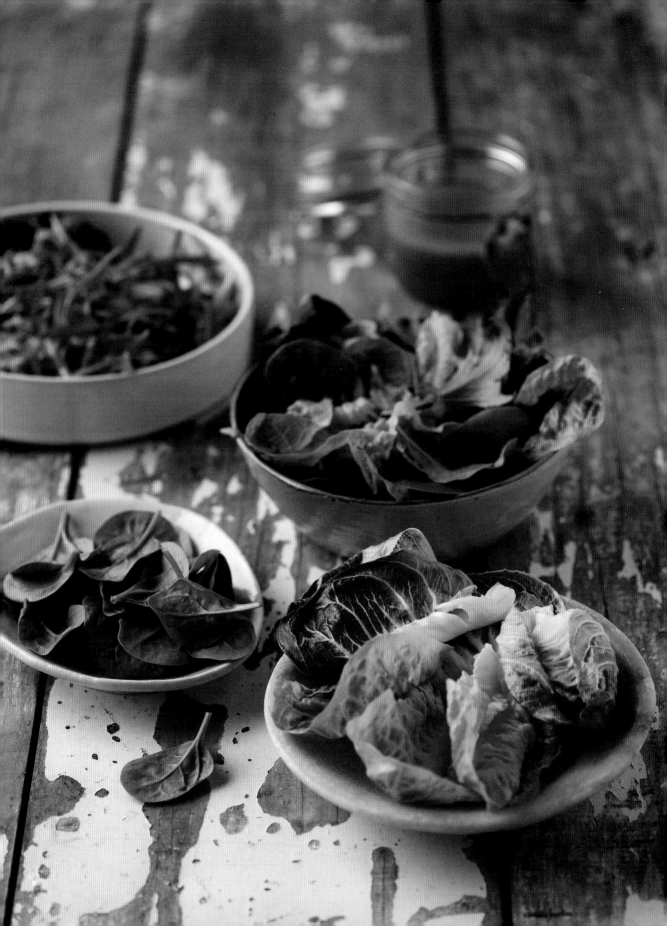

Quinoa and chicken salad

4 meals

1 x size 12 (6 lb) free-range chicken
4 quarters preserved lemon
½ teaspoon Celtic sea salt
cracked black pepper
100 g (3.75 oz) pumpkin, peeled and
    cut into 4 cm (1.5 in) chunks
2 cups hot water
½ cup quinoa
½ cup natural yoghurt
juice of 1 lime
½ Spanish onion or 2 spring onions,
    chopped
½ bunch Vietnamese mint, roughly torn
2 large handfuls baby spinach, washed
    and roughly chopped
½ cup walnuts, roughly chopped

Preheat oven to 180°C (350°F).

Prepare the chicken by patting dry with paper towel. Stuff the chicken by placing the preserved lemon quarters into the cavity. Season chicken with salt and pepper. Place chicken into an oven bag on a baking tray and roast for 1 hour.

Toss the pumpkin pieces in a splash of olive oil and add to the baking tray. Cook for approximately 15 minutes.

When the chicken is cooked, remove and set aside to cool. Once the chicken is cooled, remove skin and discard. Remove the meat from the bones and shred finely.

Place a saucepan over medium heat, add water and bring to the boil. Add quinoa and salt and cook for 10 minutes or until just tender. Take off heat, drain and rinse well under cold water. Set aside.

In a large bowl combine the natural yoghurt, onion, Vietnamese mint, baby spinach, chicken, pumpkin and quinoa. Add lime juice.

Sprinkle over walnuts and serve in bowls or place in containers to take to work.

Note: You may have pumpkin pieces already cooked and stored in the fridge. Buy a cooked chicken making this an easy salad to make.

Nutty quinoa salad

2 meals

½ cup vegetable stock
½ cup quinoa, rinsed well and drained
1 celery stick, chopped
1 spring onion, finely sliced
½ red capsicum, chopped
½ cup chopped coriander
5 mint leaves finely sliced (Vietnamese
    mint is delicious)
small handful flat-leaf parsley, finely
    chopped
¼ cup currants
¾ cup almonds, pistachios or pecans,
    roughly chopped
juice of ½ lemon or lime
15 ml (0.5 fl oz) olive oil
iceberg lettuce

Place a large saucepan of water over high heat and bring to the boil. Add stock and reduce to a simmer. Add quinoa and cook for 10 minutes or until grains are just tender. Remove from heat and drain well. Set aside to cool.

Place celery, capsicum, herbs, spring onion, currants and nuts in a bowl. Toss to combine. Dress with a squeeze of lemon or lime juice and a drizzle of oil. Serve on iceberg lettuce leaves or pack into containers to take to work.

Opposite page:
Nutty quinoa salad

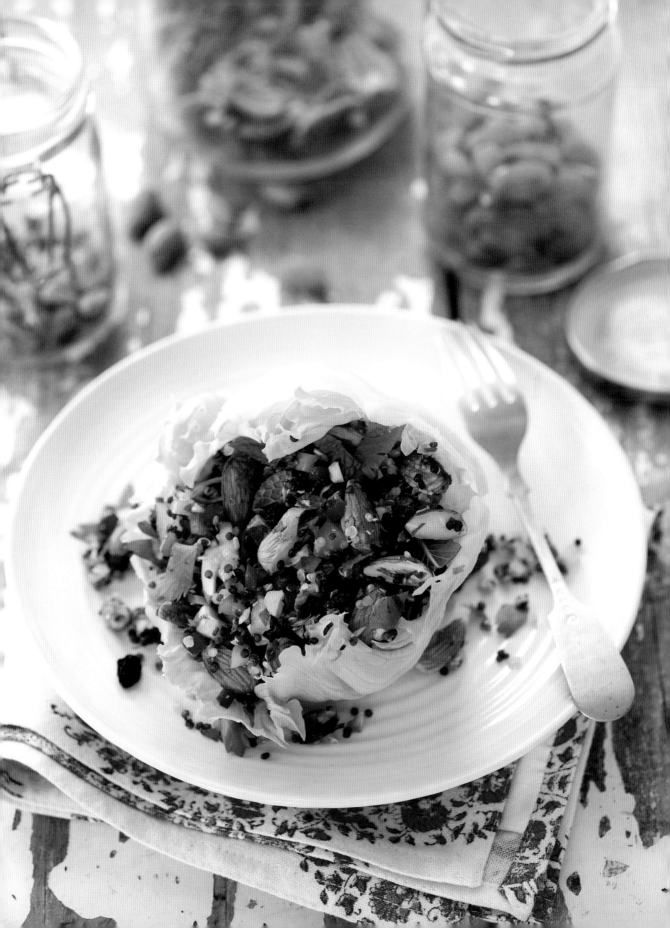

Chicken sandwich

1 meal

25 g (1 oz) goat's feta or ¼ avocado
2 slices wholegrain bread
small handful mixed salad greens,
    washed and well dried
6 cucumber slices, thinly sliced
1 tomato, thinly sliced
1 small carrot, grated
100 g (3.75 oz) cooked chicken,
    finely sliced

Spread either goat's feta or avocado on a slice of bread. Top with salad greens and thinly sliced cucumber, tomato and grated carrot. Top with chicken and finish with second slice of bread.

Tuna or salmon sandwich

1 meal

25 g (1 oz) goat's feta
2 slices wholegrain bread
small handful mixed salad greens,
    washed and well dried
1 gherkin, thinly sliced
1 tomato, thinly sliced
1 small carrot, grated
1 x 95 g (3.5 oz) can tuna or salmon,
    drained and flaked

Spread goat's feta on a slice of bread and top with salad greens, thinly sliced gherkin, tomato and grated carrot. Top with tuna or salmon and finish with second slice of bread.

Pea and spinach frittata and salad

2 meals

5 free-range or organic eggs
pinch of Celtic sea salt and cracked black
    pepper
2 tablespoons natural yoghurt
½ cup frozen peas
1 small zucchini, sliced thinly
small handful of baby spinach
2 spring onions, finely sliced
small handful mint and coriander, finely
    chopped
1 teaspoon olive oil
50 g (1.75 oz) mozzarella cheese or
    parmesan cheese, grated
salad, to serve

Preheat oven to 180°C (350°F).

In a bowl, whisk eggs and yoghurt with salt and pepper. Add peas, zucchini, baby spinach, spring onions and herbs and gently stir to combine.

Place an ovenproof, non-stick 15 cm (6 in) diameter frying pan over medium heat. Add olive oil. Pour egg mixture into pan. Sprinkle mozzarella or parmesan cheese over top.

Reduce heat to low and cook for 5 minutes. Remove and place pan in an oven and cook until set and browned on top.

Serve with a salad of your choice. One that really works is the combination of rocket, thinly sliced pear, walnuts and shaved parmesan cheese.

Opposite page: Pea and spinach frittata and salad

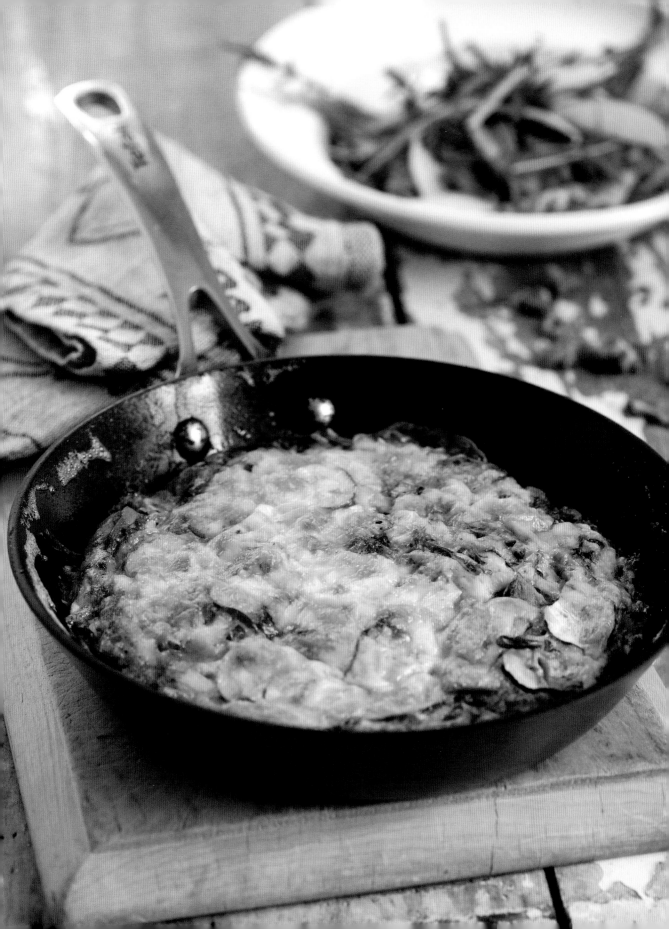

Wholemeal or spelt pasta with fresh tomato and basil sauce

Spelt pasta has more protein, amino acids, B vitamins, fibre and minerals than wheat pasta. The nutrients from spelt are absorbed quickly without making your digestive system work too hard. This makes an ideal midday meal that will give you the energy you need for the afternoon.

1 meal

100 g (3.75 oz) dried or fresh wholemeal or spelt pasta
1 teaspoon olive oil
1 small onion, finely chopped
2 cloves garlic, crushed
½ cup dry white wine
½ cup chicken or vegetable stock
2 large tomatoes, roughly chopped
fresh basil, torn into pieces
2 tablespoons parmesan cheese, grated
basil, extra to garnish

Place a large saucepan filled with water over high heat to boil. Follow the packet instructions for the time it takes to cook your preferred pasta.

Place a non-stick frying pan over medium heat, add olive oil and sauté onion and garlic for 2 minutes. Add wine and stock. Add tomatoes, reduce heat and simmer slowly uncovered for 5 minutes. Remove from heat and stir through basil.

Serve immediately over cooked spelt pasta. Garnish with parmesan cheese and extra basil.

Thai beef salad

1 meal

½ bunch fresh coriander, leaves only
½ Spanish onion, halved and finely sliced
handful rocket leaves
8 cm (3 in) piece cucumber, finely sliced
½ red chilli, deseeded and finely sliced
½ green chilli, deseeded and finely sliced
200 g (7 oz) rump steak or sirloin (trimmed of fat)
1 teaspoon olive oil
2 teaspoons brown sugar
3 tablespoons water
1 tablespoon Thai fish sauce
juice of 1 lime
3 cm (1 in) length lemongrass white part only, finely sliced

In a bowl, gently mix coriander, onion, rocket, cucumber, and chilli. Set aside.

Place a non-stick frying pan over medium-high heat. Brush the meat on both sides with olive oil. Add to pan and cook for a few minutes each side. Remove and set aside to rest.

Drain any excess fat from pan, return to heat, add sugar and water to deglaze the pan, simmer for a minute until syrupy. Remove from heat.

Add fish sauce, lime juice and lemongrass.

Thinly slice the meat, add to salad base and drizzle over sugar syrup from pan.

To serve, pile into a bowl.

Opposite page:
Thai beef salad

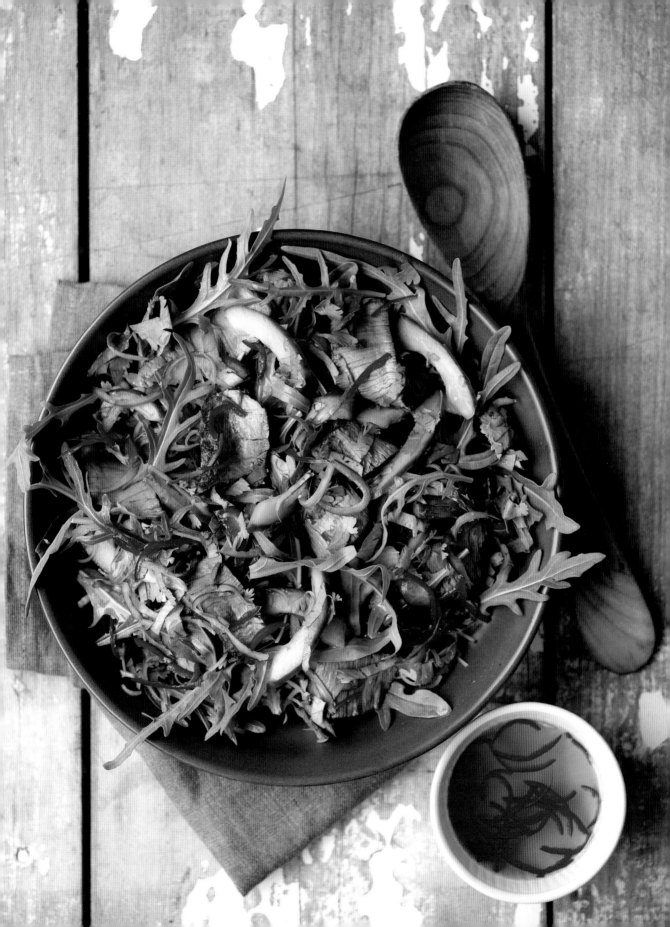

Niçoise salad

1 meal

1 free-range or organic egg
6 green beans, topped and tailed
4 cos lettuce leaves
1 tomato, cut into quarters or 4 cherry
    tomatoes halved
4 black olives
8 cm (3 in) length cucumber, sliced
1 x 95 g (3.5 oz) can tuna or salmon,
    drained and flaked
juice of $\frac{1}{2}$ a lemon
1 teaspoon olive oil
cracked black pepper

Place a saucepan filled with water over high heat and bring to the boil. Carefully lower the egg into the water with a spoon. Reduce heat and simmer for 3 minutes. Remove and run under cold water to stop the egg from cooking further. When cool, peel and cut into quarters. Blanch the beans in the hot water for 2 minutes or until just turning bright green. Remove and rinse under cold water to keep them crisp.

On serving plates, arrange the cos lettuce, tomatoes, olives, green beans, cucumber, eggs and tuna.

In a small bowl, whisk together lemon juice, oil and pepper, then drizzle over the salad. Serve immediately.

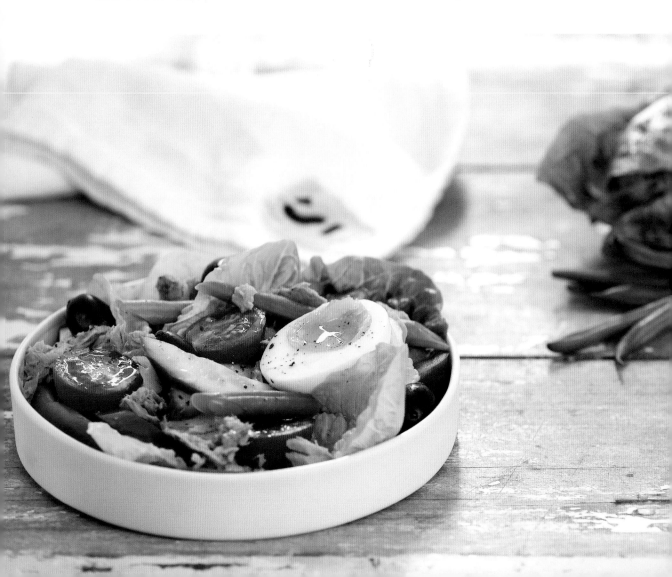

MID-AFTERNOON SNACKS

In regards to your digestive fire, if you have eaten breakfast, fruit mid-morning and a midday meal, you may not need much fuel in the afternoon. Top up your digestive fire with a small protein snack. At this time of day start reducing the carbohydrates you eat. This is only a snack so keep the quantities small.

Choose from the following list for some sustaining mid-afternoon snacks.

- 10 mixed nuts almond/pecans/walnuts/Brazil nuts and 1 fig
- 6 seaweed rice crackers with goat's feta or homemade dips
- celery and carrot sticks with goat's feta or homemade dips
- 1 hard-boiled egg
- ¼ cup natural yoghurt with berries or fruit
- 1 California roll/sushi
- protein drink
- green barley powder or spirulina mixed into apple juice
- wheat grass shot
- miso soup

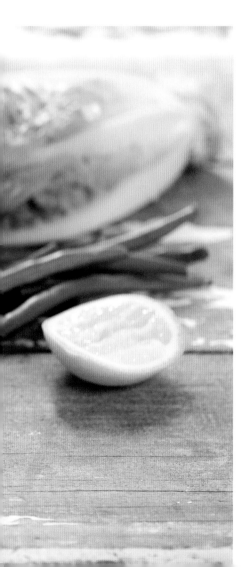

Following pages: A selection of mid-afternoon snacks

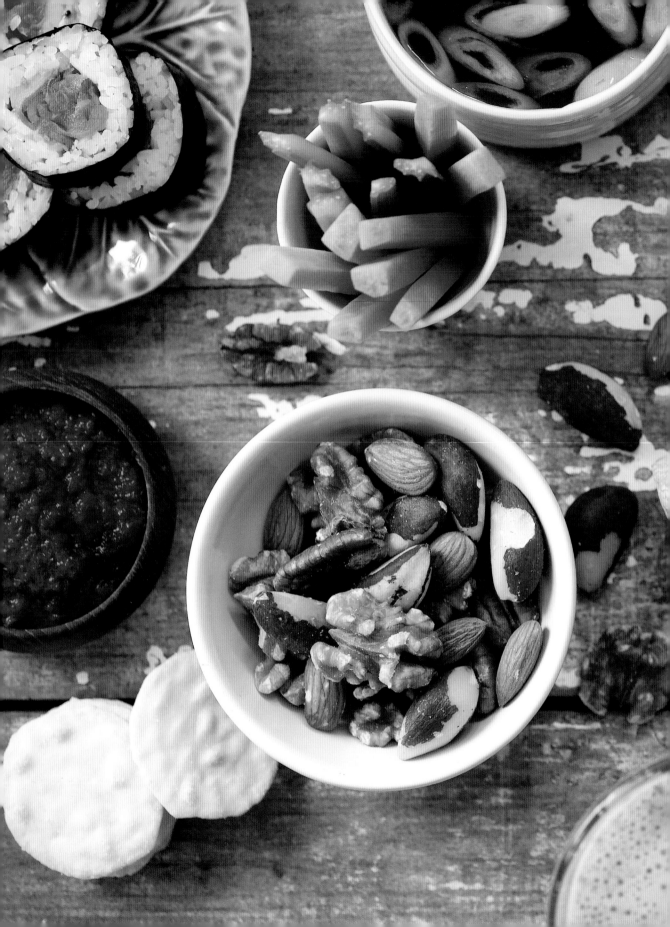

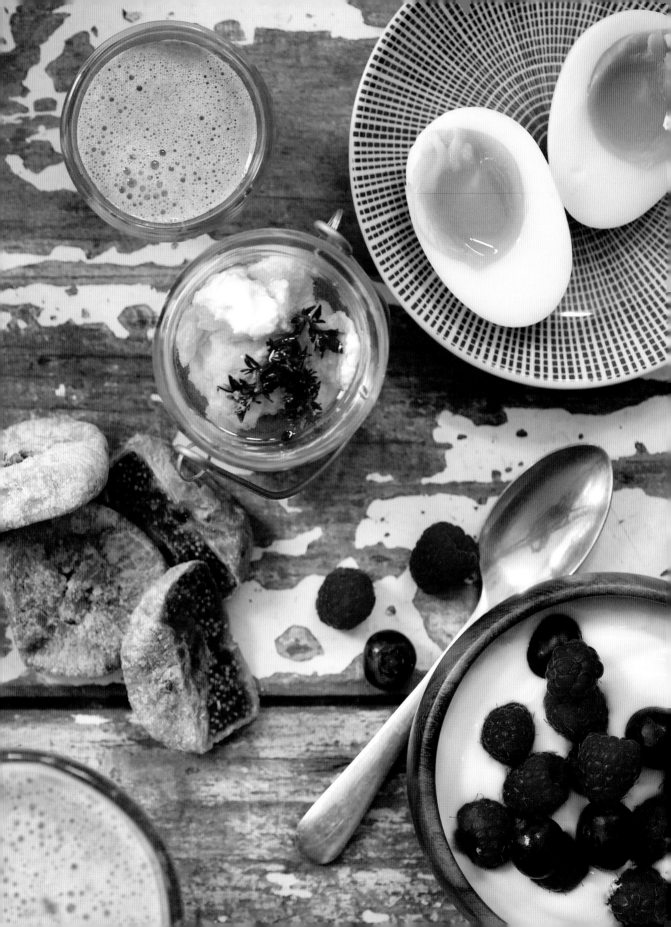

EVENING MEAL

You don't need much energy while you sleep, so your need to eat carbohydrates in the evening is low. Create your evening meal from protein and low GI foods. Protein and vegetables will provide the building blocks for your body to heal and renew while you sleep. The fibre and enzymes in salad or vegetable combinations will provide a workout for your digestive system that will get your metabolism moving.

When making your weekly meal plan choose from the following evening meals and salad accompaniments:

- 4 + 1 salads
- lean meat and 4 + 1 salad
- roasted tofu with 4 + 1 salad
- lamb cutlets with ratatouille and salad
- herb, pecan and pistachio crusted salmon with steamed green vegetables
- lemon roast chicken with salad
- warm meatball and pesto salad
- cold meat and salad
- curried chicken with warm lentil salad
- Tuscan chicken with a green salad
- chicken and vegetable bake
- osso buco with gremolata
- poached salmon salad with gherkin salsa
- spicy bean stew
- vegetable-stuffed red capsicums
- fish fillets with roasted pumpkin and green vegetables
- lamb and beans with feta and olive salsa
- stir-fried beef
- orange and ginger chicken with Asian coleslaw

Salads

Making salads interesting is easy, requiring only four ingredients as well as your choice of salad dressing.

Mix together different types of salad leaves and place in a plastic container in the refrigerator. This is then a handy and interesting salad base for many meals. Choose from:

- cos lettuce
- wild rocket
- radicchio
- watercress
- baby spinach
- endive

Salad dressing suggestions

Place ingredients in a jar with a screw-top lid and shake to combine.

- orange or mandarin juice with olive oil, honey, pinch of Celtic sea salt and Dijon mustard
- tahini, yoghurt, honey and lemon juice
- natural yoghurt with mandarin juice
- olive oil, tamari and lemon or lime juice
- natural yoghurt with freshly chopped coriander and mint

Opposite page:
Salad dressing

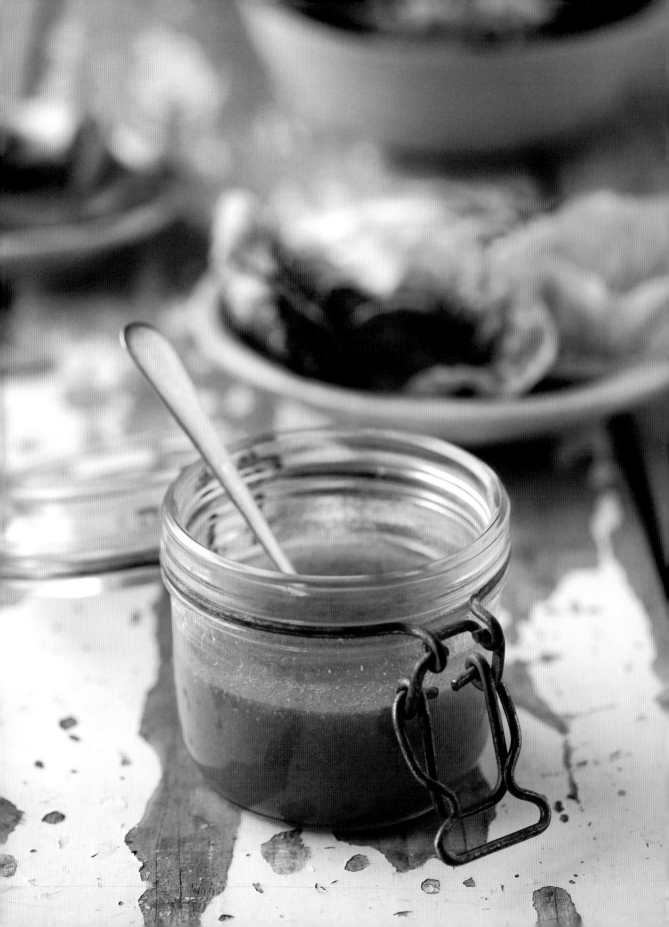

4 + 1 salads

All these salads consist of four ingredients. Simply add one of your favorite salad dressings or squeeze over fresh orange, mandarin or lemon juice. Or simply drizzle with olive oil.

- baby spinach leaves, pear slices, walnut halves, goat's feta or feta cheese
- green beans (lightly steamed), small can of butter beans, currants and walnuts
- salsa of finely chopped cucumber, gherkin, capsicum, feta cheese
- baby spinach, roasted beetroot, goat's feta and pistachios
- chopped coriander, cucumber, avocado, mint
- spanish onion, flat-leaf parsley, currants, pistachios
- layer slices of bocconcini with tomato, fresh basil leaves and drizzle with olive oil
- roasted pumpkin, baby spinach, goat's feta and walnut halves
- avocado salsa (made from avocado, coriander, cucumber, lemon juice, goat's feta)
- fresh green beans (lightly steamed), small can butter beans, snow peas, marinated goat's feta
- cherry tomatoes, bocconcini, baby spinach leaves, baby olives
- rocket leaves, pear slices, walnuts, shaved parmesan cheese
- grated beetroot, grated carrot, grated radish, chopped walnuts
- salsa of chopped cucumber, Vietnamese mint, coriander, goat's feta
- mixed green salad leaves, cucumber, celery and Vietnamese mint
- julienned snow peas, red capsicum, celery, carrot
- cucumber, tomato, kalamata olives, feta cheese
- rocket, figs, walnuts, goat's feta

Lean meat and 4 + 1 salad

This is one of the quickest and easiest meals to prepare.

1 meal

150–200 g (5.5–7 oz) of lean meat (eye fillet, porterhouse, scotch fillet or lamb steak)

olive oil

3 pieces roasted pumpkin (see p100)

4 + 1 salad of your choice (see p136)

mixed salad leaves

Place a grill plate or non-stick frying pan over high heat. Brush meat on both sides with olive oil and place in pan.

Reheat pumpkin on grill plate or pan.

While meat is cooking, prepare a 4 + 1 salad. Add roasted pumpkin and mixed salad leaves. Serve with the cooked meat.

Opposite page:
Lean meat and 4 + 1 salad

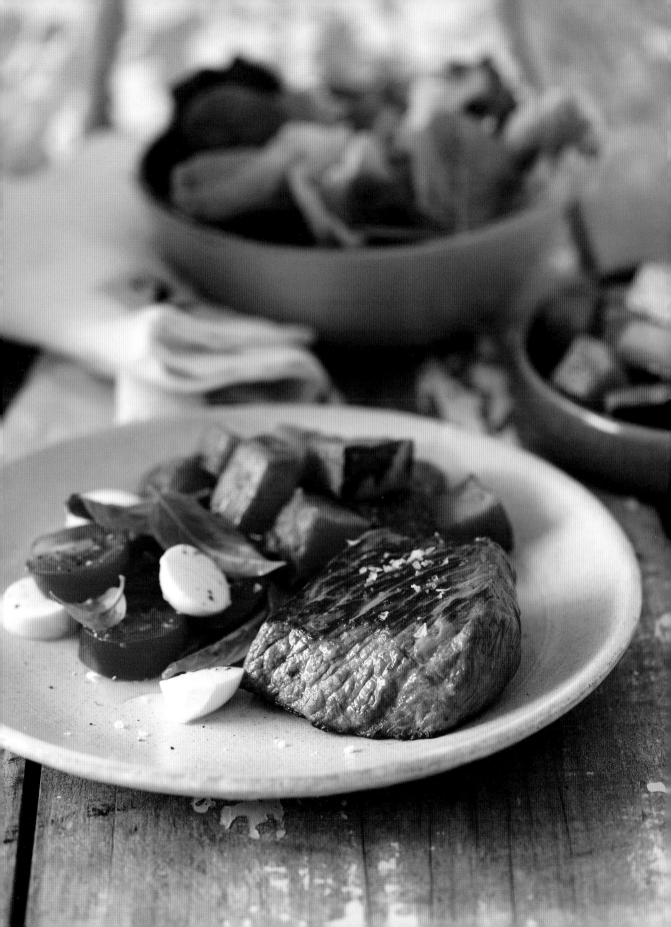

Roasted tofu with 4 + 1 salad

This salad needs to be prepared the night before.

1 meal

250 g (8.75 oz) firm tofu
1 tablespoon olive oil
4 tablespoons tamari
¾ cup orange juice
1 teaspoon sweet chilli sauce
1 teaspoon grated ginger
1 tablespoon lemon juice

4 + 1 salad of your choice (see p136) or steamed green vegetables, to serve

Slice tofu into 4 pieces, crossways. Place a non-stick frying pan over high heat, add oil and tofu and fry until brown on all sides. Remove and place tofu in a small baking dish.

In a small bowl, combine tamari, orange juice, sweet chilli sauce, ginger and lemon juice and pour over the tofu. Allow it to marinate for 2 hours or ideally overnight.

Preheat oven to 180°C (350°F). Bake tofu until the marinade reduces down to a sticky sauce. This will take approximately 40 minutes. Serve warm with your choice of 4 + 1 salad or steamed green vegetables.

Lamb cutlets with ratatouille and salad

1 meal and enough ratatouille to add as a salad to another 2 meals

For the ratatouille

1 teaspoon olive oil
1 small Spanish onion, finely diced
2 garlic cloves, crushed
1 red capsicum, cut into 2 cm dice
1 green capsicum, cut into 2 cm dice
2 large ripe tomatoes, cut into 2 cm dice
1 small eggplant, cut into 2 cm dice
1 small zucchini, cut into 2 cm dice
pinch of Celtic sea salt
½ teaspoon favorite spice mix (see p95)
1 tablespoon tomato paste
2 tablespoons white wine
Sprig of thyme or 6 basil leaves or a
    rosemary flavour bag
1 tablespoon olive oil, extra for basting
½ teaspoon cumin for basting
150 g (5.5 oz) lamb cutlets (3 or 4 small)
small handful flat-leaf parsley, roughly
    chopped
mixed salad greens and your favorite
    dressing, to serve

Place a large deep-sided frying pan or wok over medium high heat. Add oil and sauté the onions and garlic for 3 minutes.

Add the capsicum and cook for another 2 minutes. Add tomatoes, eggplant, zucchini, salt, favorite spice mix, tomato paste, white wine and your choice of herbs. Reduce heat and cook gently for 15 minutes.

Place a grill plate over high heat. Combine olive oil and cumin and brush mixture over the lamb cutlets. Place on grill and cook for 2 minutes each side. Remove and set aside to rest.

To serve, place half a cup of ratatouille in the centre of a plate and arrange lamb cutlets on top. Sprinkle with chopped parsley.

Serve with a salad of mixed salad leaves and your favorite dressing.

Note: Ratatouille is great as a cold salad with frittata for lunch.

Herb, pecan and pistachio crusted salmon with steamed green vegetables

This meal is high in essential fatty acids. The salmon is very filling and satisfying because of this.

1 meal

5 pecans
5 pistachio nuts, unsalted
1 slice stale bread
1 teaspoon pesto (see p98)
180 g (6.5 oz) salmon steak
A selection of your favorite green vegetables (for example, 1 piece broccoli, 6 green beans, 6 slices zucchini, 6 sugar snap peas, 1 small bok choy)
Half an orange or mandarin

Preheat oven to 180° C (350°F).

Place nuts and stale bread in a food processor and process until they resemble fine breadcrumbs. Combine with pesto and coat the salmon with this paste.

Place salmon on baking tray lined with baking paper and bake for approximately six to ten minutes depending on how pink you like your salmon.

Lightly steam the green vegetables. Drizzle steamed greens with orange or mandarin juice and serve with salmon.

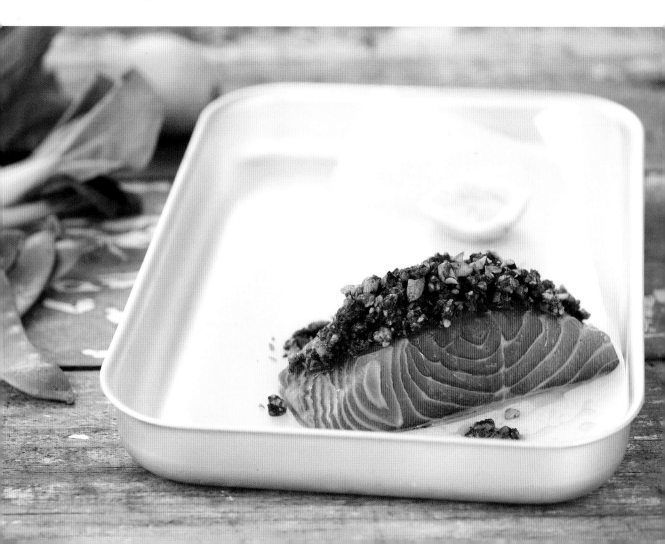

Lemon roast chicken with salad

4 meals

1 x size 12 (6 lb) free-range chicken
4 pieces preserved lemon
1 onion, peeled and halved
1 oven baking bag
4 + 1 salad (see p136)
4 pieces roasted pumpkin (see p100)
A small handful of mixed salad leaves

Preheat oven to 180°C (350°F).

Pat chicken dry with a paper towel. Rub a preserved lemon quarter over the skin of the chicken and then place all the lemon pieces inside the cavity along with onion.

Place chicken in an oven bag and onto a baking tray. Tie the top of the bag and make a couple of holes for the steam to escape. Bake for 1 hour or until the chicken is cooked.

Serve with a 4 + 1 salad, roasted pumpkin and mixed salad leaves. Any leftover chicken can be used in mountain bread wraps or as a meal salad for lunch.

Warm meatball and pesto salad

1 meal

150–200 g (5.5–7 oz) lean minced beef
½ teaspoon favorite spice mix (see p95)
½ small onion, finely chopped
1 clove garlic, crushed
1 teaspoon olive oil
A small handful of mixed salad leaves
4 cherry tomatoes
6 cm (2.5 in) piece cucumber, thinly sliced
4 sugar snap peas
6 slices red capsicum
2 teaspoons pesto per serving (see p98)

In a bowl, combine minced beef, favorite spice mix, onion and garlic. Using your hands make small walnut-sized meatballs.

Place a non-stick frying pan over medium heat, add olive oil and cook the meatballs, browning them on all sides.

In a small bowl, combine mixed salad leaves, cherry tomatoes, cucumber, capsicum and sugar snap peas. Add meatballs and toss gently with a dollop of pesto.

Cold meat and salad

A quick and easy meal is cold meat that you may have left over or you can buy cooked slices of chicken, turkey, lamb or beef and make a 4 + 1 salad (see p136) with your choice of mixed salad leaves.

Opposite page: Warm meatball and pesto salad

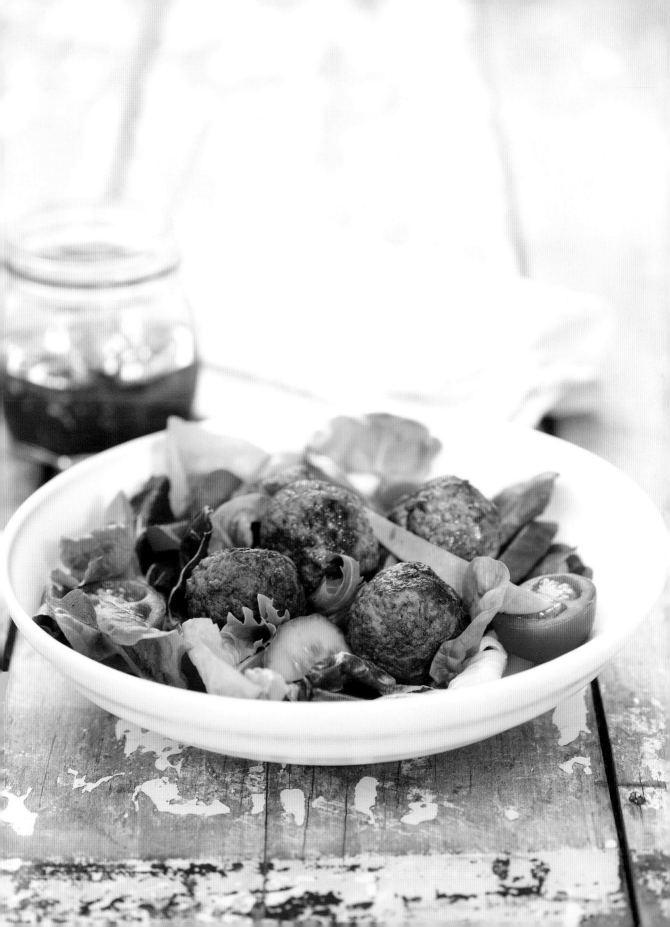

Beef with oyster sauce

1 meal

150–200 g (5.5–7 oz) rump steak cut
    into thin strips
1 teaspoon olive oil
1 clove garlic, crushed
handful of snow peas
handful of green beans
½ red capsicum, thinly sliced
2 spring onions, thinly sliced
1 tablespoon oyster sauce
½ tablespoon Thai fish sauce
1 tablespoon sweet chilli sauce
1 bunch bok choy, washed and leaves
    separated
½ bunch Chinese broccoli, washed and
    cut into large pieces
coriander, finely chopped

Place a non-stick frying pan or wok over
high heat. Add steak, oil and garlic and
stir-fry for 2 minutes. Add snow peas, green
beans, red capsicum, spring onion, oyster
sauce, Thai fish sauce, chilli sauce and stir
fry for 2 minutes.

Add bok choy and Chinese broccoli, cover
with lid and steam for 2 minutes.

To serve, place steamed Chinese broccoli
and bok choy in a bowl and serve meat on
top. Sprinkle with coriander.

Note: A quarter of a cup of quinoa cooked
in 2 cups of hot water can be added to this
meal if you feel that you need something
more substantial.

Curried chicken with warm lentil salad

1 meal and enough lentil salad to add to
another 2 meals

200 g (7 oz) chicken breast
1 tablespoon red curry paste
2 cups water
½ cup chicken or vegetable stock
½ cup brown lentils
1 teaspoon olive oil
1 spring onion, finely chopped
1 small carrot, finely diced
1 celery stalk, finely diced
1 small red capsicum, deseeded and
    finely diced
¼ cup coriander or flat-leaf parsley, finely
    chopped
1 red or green chilli, deseeded and finely
    sliced
drizzle of olive oil
squeeze of lime or lemon juice
flat-leaf parsley, roughly chopped

Rub chicken breast with red curry paste,
place on a plate and marinate in fridge for a
few hours or overnight.

Place a saucepan over high heat, add water
and stock and bring to boil. Add lentils and
cook for 20 minutes or until tender. Remove
from heat and drain well.

Place a non-stick frying pan over medium
heat, add olive oil. Place chicken breast in
pan and cook for 5 minutes each side.

In a small bowl, combine lentils, spring
onions, vegetables, coriander and chilli.
Drizzle over olive oil and lime or lemon juice.

To serve, place half a cup of lentil salad in
the middle of a serving plate and top with a
chicken breast. Garnish with parsley.

Tuscan chicken with a green salad

1 meal

1 teaspoon olive oil
1 small Spanish onion, finely chopped
1 clove garlic, crushed
200 g (7 oz) chicken breast, cut into 4 pieces
¼ cup dry white wine
¼ cup kalamata olives, pitted and chopped
200 g (7 oz) diced tomatoes (place the balance from a 400–425g (14.5–15 oz) can in a clip lock bag and freeze for another use)
½ teaspoon favorite spice mix (see p95)
large handful flat-leaf parsley, roughly chopped
4 + 1 salad (see p136) or mixed salad greens with your favorite dressing

Place a non-stick frying pan with a tight fitting lid over medium heat. Add olive oil. Gently sauté onion and garlic for 3 minutes. Add chicken pieces and brown evenly. Add white wine, olives, diced tomatoes and spice mix.

Reduce heat and simmer covered for 20 minutes or until chicken is tender. Serve chicken sprinkled with chopped parsley and a 4 + 1 salad or mixed salad greens with your favorite dressing.

Chicken and vegetable bake

If you have a slow cooker or crockpot this can be made in the morning and cook through the day. Your kitchen will smell very inviting as you arrive home at the end of a busy day.

2 meals

1 teaspoon olive oil
2 cloves garlic, minced
1 carrot, finely diced
1 parsnip, finely diced
8 cm (3 in) piece sweet potato, finely diced
1 celery stalk, finely diced
1 leek, white part only, finely diced
400 g (14.5 oz) chicken thigh fillets, skin off and fat trimmed
1 small potato, grated (there is a lot of nourishment in the skin so use it all)
1 cup chicken stock
¼ cup dry white wine
2 dried bay leaves
¼ cup flat leaf parsley, finely chopped
steamed green vegetables or mixed leaf salad, to serve

Preheat oven to 180°C (350°F).

Place a large non-stick frying pan over medium heat. Add oil, garlic and vegetables and sauté for 3 minutes. Remove and place in lidded casserole dish.

Place chicken pieces in pan and brown on all sides. Remove and add to casserole dish.

Add stock, white wine, bay leaves and grated potato and cover.

Bake for an hour or until chicken is tender and sauce has thickened. Garnish with parsley.

Serve with steamed green vegetables or a mixed leaf salad.

Osso buco with gremolata

2 meals

1 teaspoon olive oil
1 onion, finely chopped
2 cloves garlic, finely chopped
1 large carrot, diced
1 large celery stalk, diced
½ cup dry white wine
1 teaspoon olive oil, extra
2 x 250 g (8.75 oz) osso buco steaks
1 heaped teaspoon tomato paste
1½ cups beef stock
2 cups hot water

1 rosemary flavour bag (see p96)
1 teaspoon favorite spice mix (see p95)
1 small potato, grated (there is a lot of nourishment in the skin so use it all)

For the gremolata

large handful of flat-leaf parsley, finely chopped
1 clove garlic, crushed
1 lemon, grated zest only
A selection of your favorite green vegetables (for example, 1 piece broccoli, 6 green beans, 6 slices zucchini, 6 sugar snap peas, 1 small bok choy), to serve

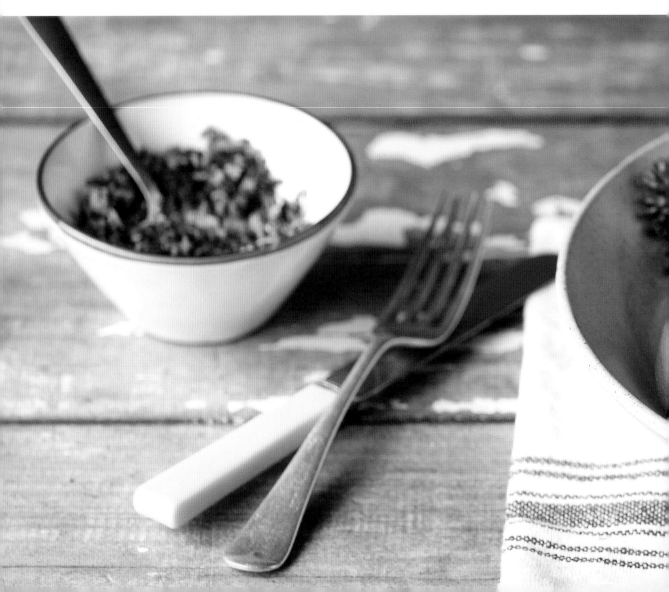

Preheat oven to 180°C (350°F).

Place a non-stick frying pan over medium heat. Add olive oil, onion and garlic and sauté for 1 minute. Add carrot and celery and stir to soften for another minute. Add dry white wine and cook for another minute.

Remove from heat and transfer to a lidded casserole dish. Return the non-stick frying pan to medium heat, add extra olive oil and the meat and brown. Remove and add to casserole dish along with tomato paste, beef stock, hot water, rosemary flavour bag and favorite spice mix. Add a grated potato, which will provide the starch to thicken the stew.

Bake in the oven for 2 hours or until beef is very tender. Remove the lid and bake for a further 30 minutes to thicken the sauce.

To make the gremolata, combine all the ingredients in a small bowl. It will add tang and raw enzymes to your osso buco. Prepare and steam your vegetables.

Remove the casserole from the oven, take out the rosemary flavour bag, serve sprinkled with gremolata and serve with the steamed green vegetables.

Note: The marrow in the osso buco bones is high in iron and minerals so make sure you eat it!

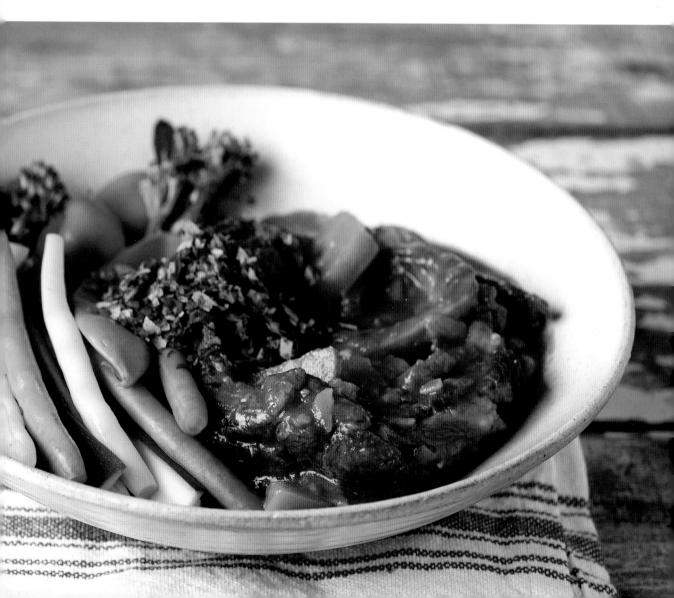

Poached salmon with gherkin salsa

1 meal

¼ cup dry white wine
1 cup water
150–180 g (5.5–6.5 oz) salmon steak
slice lemon
sprig coriander

For gherkin salsa

1 large sweet gherkin, finely diced
1 celery stick, finely diced
coriander leaves, finely chopped
1 tablespoon goat's feta
squeeze of lemon juice
mixed salad leaves
4 cherry tomatoes, cut in half

Place a large saucepan over low heat. Add wine and water and bring to a slow simmer. Place salmon, lemon and coriander in pan and poach, covered, for 5 minutes.

In a small bowl, combine gherkin, celery, coriander, goat's feta and lemon juice. Arrange mixed salad leaves on a serving plate.

Remove salmon and flake into pieces. Place on mixed salad leaves, top with gherkin salsa and cherry tomatoes.

Spicy bean stew

2 meals

½ cup dried kidney beans (soaked overnight in water, well drained)
½ cup dried chickpeas (soaked overnight in water, well drained)
1 teaspoon olive oil
1 small Spanish onion, finely diced
1 small carrot, roughly chopped
8 cm (3 in) piece sweet potato, roughly chopped
1 red capsicum, roughly chopped
1 clove garlic, crushed
1 small red or green chilli, deseeded and thinly sliced
1 teaspoon favorite spice mix (see p95)
1 rosemary flavour bag (see p96)
1 x 400–425g (14.5–15 oz) can diced tomatoes
1½ cups vegetable stock
1 teaspoon tomato paste
10 fresh green beans, cut into 3 cm pieces
¼ cup flat-leaf parsley, roughly chopped

Place the kidney beans and chickpeas in a large saucepan. Cover with water, simmer uncovered for 20 minutes. Drain and cool.

Place a large heavy-based frying pan over medium heat. Add olive oil, onion, carrot, sweet potato, capsicum, garlic and chilli and sauté for a couple of minutes. Stir in the favorite spice mix and simmer for another minute.

Add the beans, chickpeas, tomatoes, rosemary flavour bag, vegetable stock and tomato paste. Simmer uncovered for an hour or until the beans and vegetables are tender.

Remove rosemary flavour bag, add the fresh green beans and cook for another couple of minutes. Just before serving sprinkle with parsley.

Serve with mixed salad leaves and your favorite salad dressing.

Note: A simple and tasty serving idea is to crumble 50 g (1.75 oz) of feta cheese or goat's feta into the parsley, combine well and spoon over the top.

Vegetable-stuffed red capsicums

Prepare the cooked rice for your filling beforehand in this easy to prepare recipe.

2 meals

1 teaspoon olive oil

½ onion, finely chopped

1 clove garlic, crushed

1 ripe tomato, roughly chopped

6 cm (2.5 in) piece of zucchini, finely chopped

10 cm (4 in) piece celery, finely chopped

½ teaspoon favorite spice mix (see p95)

1 teaspoon tomato paste

1 cup vegetable or beef stock

½ cup cooked basmati rice

½ x 400–425g (14.5–15 oz) can kidney beans, drained and well rinsed. The other half can be put in a zip lock bag and used in a salad or another meal.

¼ cup parsley, roughly chopped

½ cup feta cheese, crumbled or cut into small cubes

2 large red capsicums, slice off the tops, remove seeds and membranes

Mixed salad leaves, sliced cucumber and your favorite dressing, to serve

Preheat oven to 350°F (180C). Place a non-stick frying pan over medium heat. Add oil, onions and garlic and sauté for a few minutes. Add tomatoes, zucchini, celery, favorite spice mix, tomato paste and stock. Cook for 10 minutes then remove from heat.

Add the kidney beans, cooked rice, chopped parsley and feta cheese.

Spoon the mixture into the capsicums and place the capsicum lid on top. Place on a lined baking tray. Bake in a moderate oven for 40 to 45 minutes or until the capsicums are soft. While these bake your kitchen will smell delicious.

Note: If you would like to add more substance to this meal then serve with some baked pumpkin.

Another simple option is to stuff the red capsicums with leftover bolognaise sauce that you have cooked for the kids. Add a small can of drained and well-rinsed kidney beans, top with a little grated cheddar cheese and bake.

Fish fillets with roasted pumpkin and green vegetables

1 meal

3 small pieces roasted pumpkin (see p100)

8 green beans

8 sugar snap peas

1 teaspoon olive oil

200 g (7 oz) flathead

flat-leaf parsley or coriander, roughly chopped

¼ lemon, for squeezing

Preheat oven to 300°F (150°C) to reheat roast pumpkin. Cook beans for 2 minutes, then add sugar snap peas and cook for another 2 minutes.

Place a non-stick frying pan over medium-heat, add olive oil and fish fillets, cooking for about 2 minutes each side or until the fish flakes.

On a serving plate, place the pumpkin, then beans and sugar snap peas and top with fish fillets and sprinkle over parsley or coriander. Add a squeeze of lemon juice and serve immediately.

Lamb and beans with feta and olive salsa

1 meal

200 g (7 oz) lamb back straps or lamb steaks

1 teaspoon olive oil

sprig of rosemary

1 clove garlic, crushed

½ Spanish onion, finely diced

¼ cup small black olives, pitted and finely diced

¼ small red capsicum, finely diced

50 g (1.75 oz) goat's feta, crumbled

large handful green beans, topped and tailed

½ x 400 g (14.5 oz) can butter beans, drained and well rinsed. The other half can be put in a zip-lock bag and used in a salad or another meal.

¼ cup flat-leaf parsley, roughly chopped

mixed salad greens and your favorite dressing, to serve

Place meat in a zip-lock bag with olive oil, rosemary and garlic. Seal bag and marinate for at least a couple of hours. Ideally you would prepare this meat on your shopping day so it is ready in advance.

In a small bowl, combine onion, olives, red capsicum and goat's feta.

Place a grill plate or non-stick frying pan over high heat. Remove meat from marinade and place on grill. Cook for 2 minutes each side. Remove and set aside to rest. Steam the green beans for 2 minutes.

To serve, slice the meat thinly and layer the plate with the meat, beans and the salsa. Sprinkle with parsley.

Serve with mixed salad leaves and your favorite dressing.

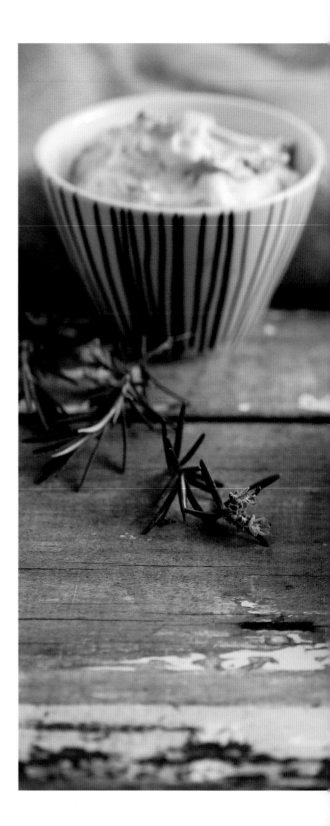

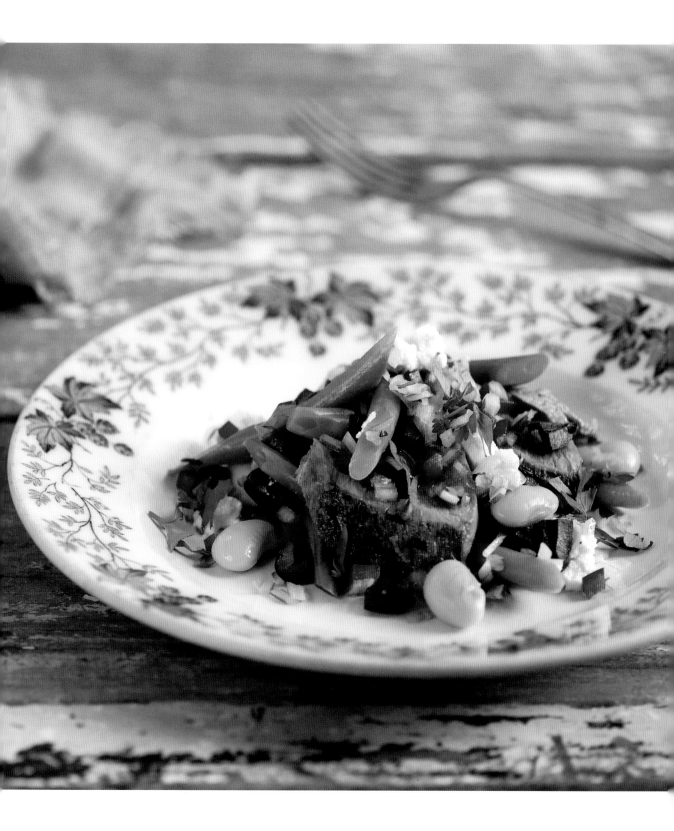

Stir-fried beef

1 meal

If you marinate the meat on shopping day it will be well marinated and ready for you to prepare.

1 teaspoon olive oil
2 cloves garlic, crushed
1 teaspoon grated ginger
150–200 g (5.5–7 oz) rump steak sliced into thin strips
½ Spanish onion, finely sliced
½ red capsicum, deseeded and finely sliced
3 small mushrooms, finely sliced
4 sugar snap peas
6 green beans
1 baby bok choy, leaves separated
1 bunch broccolini, stems trimmed
small handful coriander leaves, finely chopped

Place meat in a zip lock bag with olive oil, garlic and ginger. Seal bag and marinate for at least a couple of hours or overnight.

Place a non-stick frying pan or wok over high heat. Add meat and marinade and cook meat quickly, until just cooked through. Remove and set aside in a warm place. Add onion, red capsicum and mushrooms and cook for 2 minutes, stirring occasionally.

Add the snap peas, green beans, bok choy and broccolini and cook for a minute or two. Return meat to pan and mix well, reheating meat.

Serve sprinkled with coriander.

Note: A quarter of a cup of quinoa cooked in 2 cups of hot water can be added to this meal if you feel that you need something more substantial.

Orange and ginger chicken with Asian coleslaw

1 meal (note: there will be enough salad left over to have as a midday meal with a can of tuna or salmon)

For the Asian coleslaw

½ cup finely shredded red cabbage
½ cup finely shredded Chinese cabbage
1 small carrot, julienned
1 spring onion, cut on the diagonal into 3 cm (1 in) pieces
5 Vietnamese mint leaves, torn
handful coriander leaves
small handful chopped walnuts
4 sugar snap peas, thinly sliced

1 teaspoon olive oil
200 g (7 oz) free-range or organic chicken breast, skin removed
1 teaspoon grated ginger
juice of two oranges
2 tablespoons tamari
2 teaspoons sweet chilli sauce

In a large serving bowl, combine all the coleslaw ingredients. Cover and set aside in a cool place.

Place a non-stick pan over medium heat. Add olive oil and chicken and brown on both sides. Add ginger, orange juice, tamari and sweet chilli sauce. Reduce heat and simmer covered for about 5 minutes or until chicken is almost cooked. Remove lid and cook until sauce thickens. Add more orange juice if the sauce thickens before the chicken is cooked.

To serve, slice the chicken into four pieces and serve with salad. Pour over the pan juices and serve immediately.

Opposite page: Orange and ginger chicken with Asian coleslaw

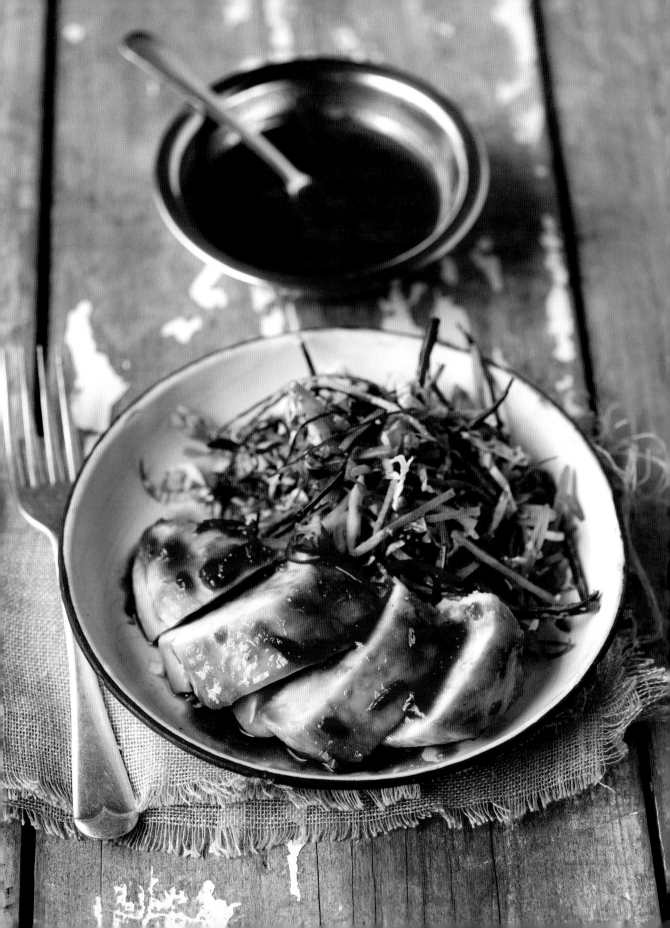

SWEET TREATS AND TEA

Having nourishing meals means that you will not crave sugar for an energy boost. When your body is nourished, an occasional sweet treat becomes a delight rather than a choice that will leave you feeling guilty.

Some people really look forward to having a treat after their evening meal. If this is really important to you then choose a treat that also has ingredients that offer nourishment. Because most sweet treats contain some carbohydrates your treat is best eaten during the day so that you can burn off the carbohydrates well before sleeping. Consider having a treat as your afternoon snack rather than having it at night.

Some sweet treat suggestions include:

• Flourless chocolate cake
• Flourless orange cake
• Muesli bars with dates
• Honeyed yoghurt with fresh berries and almonds
• Baked ricotta cake
• Soy ice-cream with chopped nuts

Flourless chocolate cake

This cake is very rich, so a small slice is very satisfying. This cake can be sliced into 8 to 10 portion-controlled pieces and frozen.

4 free-range or organic eggs, separated
150 g (5.5 oz) dark chocolate, melted
⅓ cup cocoa, sifted
⅓ cup hot water
125 g (4.5 oz) butter, melted and cooled slightly
1 cup raw sugar
2 cups almond meal
icing sugar, for dusting

Preheat oven to 180°C (350°F). Grease and line a 20–22 cm (8–9 in) round springform cake tin.

In a small bowl, lightly beat egg yolks. In another bowl, beat egg whites until soft peaks form.

Place chocolate in a heatproof bowl and place over a saucepan of simmering water. Stir the chocolate until it's melted.

In a small bowl, combine cocoa with hot water and mix until smooth.

In a large mixing bowl combine melted butter, sugar and almond meal and stir until combined. Gradually add egg yolks, mixing well after each addition. Add the cocoa paste along with the melted chocolate. Stir until smooth. Gently fold in egg whites.

Pour mixture into prepared tin and bake for an hour. Test with a skewer. When skewer comes out clean cake is cooked. Cool in tin.

Gently turn out onto a serving plate and dust with icing sugar.

Opposite page:
Flourless chocolate cake

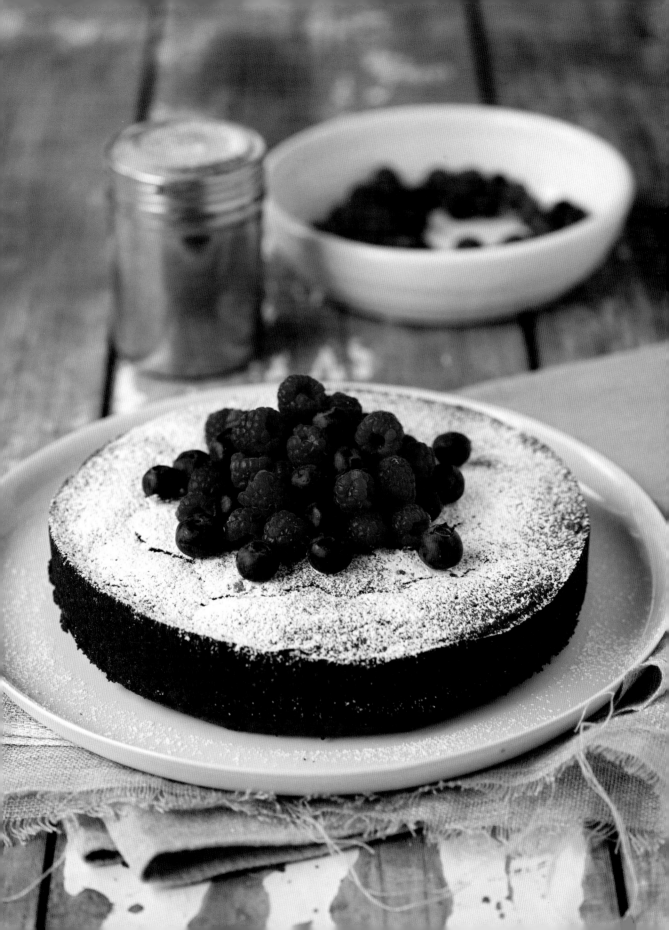

Flourless orange cake

This cake can be sliced into 8 to 10 portion-controlled pieces and frozen.

1 large sweet orange or 3 small mandarins
3 free-range or organic eggs
1 cup raw sugar
2 cups almond meal
½ teaspoon baking powder
icing sugar, for dusting

Preheat oven to 180°C (350°F). Grease and line a 20–22 cm (8–9 in) round springform cake tin.

Place a large saucepan over medium heat, fill with water, add orange or mandarins and boil for about 30 minutes. Remove fruit, drain and allow to cool.

Halve the fruit and remove any seeds. Add fruit and skin to a food processor and blend until smooth.

In a large bowl, beat eggs and sugar until pale and thick.

Gently stir in almond meal, baking powder and pureed fruit until well combined.

Pour mixture into the prepared pan and bake for 50 to 60 minutes. Test cake with a skewer. If the skewer comes out clean, the cake is cooked. Cool in the tin. Gently turn out onto a serving plate and dust with icing sugar.

Note: Add 1 tablespoon of rosewater to the fruit when it's cooking to give a Middle Eastern flavour. You can also sprinkle some almond meal into the tin to stop the cake from sticking.

Muesli bars with dates

Cut into 10 slices. Place in zip-lock bags and freeze.

2 cups rolled oats
¼ cup sesame seeds
¾ cup dates, roughly chopped
¼ cup dried apricots, roughly chopped
½ cup pecans, roughly chopped
½ cup raw sugar
2 eggs, lightly beaten
½ cup grapeseed oil or light olive oil

Preheat oven to 180°C (350°F). Grease and line a 25 cm x 15 cm (10 in x 6 in) baking tin.

In a large mixing bowl, combine oats, sesame seeds, dates, apricots, raw sugar and pecans. Add eggs and oil and mix well.

Press mixture into prepared tin and bake for 30 minutes or until slightly browned. Place a piece of baking paper over tin to stop the top from browning too quickly. Remove from oven and cool completely before cutting into bars.

Honeyed yoghurt with fresh berries and almonds

½ teaspoon honey
½ cup natural yoghurt
½ cup of mixed berries (strawberries, raspberries, blueberries)
6 almonds, roughly chopped

Stir honey through the yoghurt and place in a serving bowl.

Top with the mixed berries and chopped nuts.

Opposite page: Honeyed yoghurt with fresh berries and almonds

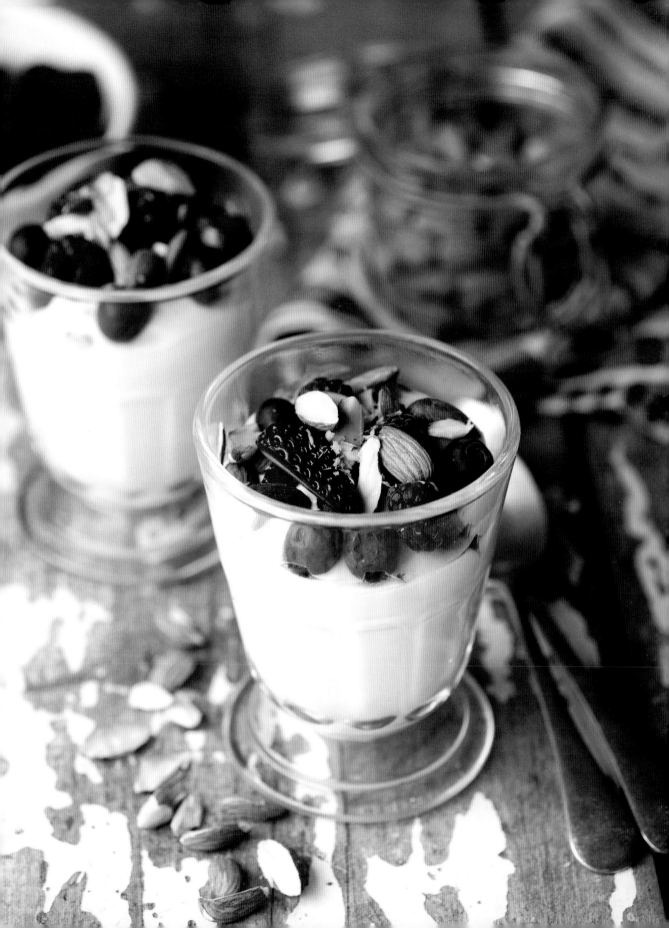

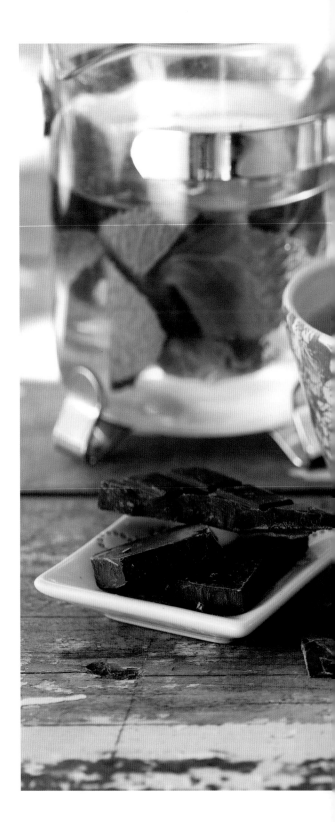

Baked ricotta cake

This cake can be sliced into 8 to 10 portion-controlled pieces and frozen.

¼ cup castor sugar
4 free-range or organic eggs
¼ teaspoon vanilla essence or ½ vanilla bean
1 kg (2.2 lbs) ricotta, beaten until smooth
¼ cup honey
juice of 1 lemon and finely grated zest
¼ cup currants soaked in 1 cup of jasmine-scented green tea or Earl Grey tea for 30 minutes
icing sugar, for dusting

Preheat oven to 180°C (350°F). Grease and line a 8–9 in (20-22 cm) round springform cake tin.

Place sugar and eggs in a large bowl or food processor and beat well for 3 minutes.

Add vanilla essence or split vanilla bean and scrape into egg mixture. Add ricotta, honey, lemon zest, and lemon juice and mix gently for 2 minutes.

Drain the currants and fold into the mixture.

Pour the batter into the prepared pan and bake for 60 minutes or until golden. Allow the cake to slowly cool in tin.

Remove the side of the springform tin and place cake on a plate. Dust with icing sugar and serve.

Tea

Visit tea shops and try different leaf tea blends. Leaf teas can have therapeutic properties and add a zing to your tastebuds. Buy a teapot and experiment. You can add your own flavourings such as mint leaves; ginger slices; lemon juice and honey; liquorice root and peppermint; green tea and lemongrass and ginger.

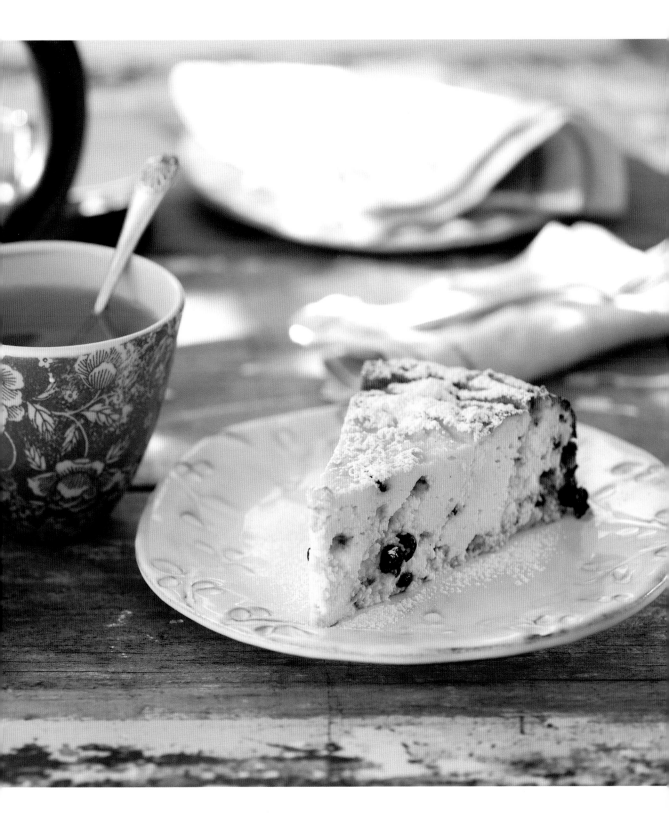

Soy ice-cream with chopped nuts

1 meal

1 scoop chocolate soy ice-cream
6 almonds or pecans, roughly chopped
plain ice-cream cone

Place chopped nuts on a saucer.
Place a scoop of soy ice-cream in cone and
roll the ice-cream in the nuts.

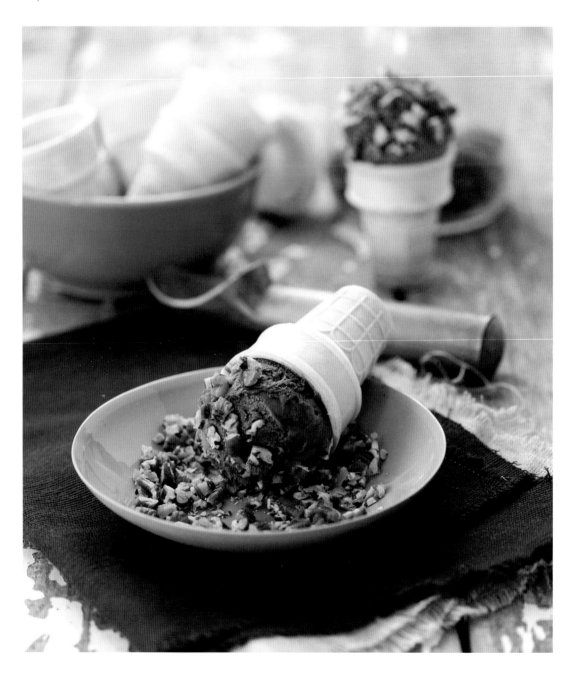

Eating out

Eating out is enjoyable and a great way to share time with family and friends. While you are working towards your weight loss and wellness goals you can still live a little and go out for dinner. There are healthy choices that you can make, however, so you can have your cake with friends or go out for a meal and still be on track to attain your weight loss goals.

Following are some ideas to help you in your choices.

- When you eat out, always choose the smaller portion on offer.
- Order meat and salad with no chips or potatoes. This could be a piece of steak, a chicken breast or a piece of fish.
- Order Thai beef salad or a chicken salad.
- When ordering a salad of any kind, ask for the salad dressing to be served on the side. If you choose to use the dressing, you can control the amount. Salad dressings can carry a lot of fat and calories if you don't know what is in them.
- For breakfast, order poached eggs instead of fried eggs and replace the bacon with tomatoes, mushrooms and spinach. Leave out the hash browns.
- Request wholegrain breads.
- Say no to soft drink (soda) with your meals. Drink plain water if you are thirsty.
- Choose broth soups rather than creamy soups that are high in calories and bad fats.
- Ask for chopped parsley sprinkled over cooked food to add some enzymes to your meal.

Choices for eating out include:

- Vietnamese restaurants serve lots of salads and use fresh herbs to flavour meals.
- Japanese restaurants have miso soup, teriyaki chicken or beef and salmon dishes, along with sushi that is a low-fat option. Avoid deep-fried foods and order steamed rice rather than fried.
- Italian restaurants are good for meat and salad but pass on pizza and pasta.
- Greek restaurants offer seafood and lamb with fresh Greek salads.

For quick snacks on the run, buy a packet of mixed unsalted nuts, a protein drink, two pieces of fruit or fruit salad, California rolls, sushi, a freshly made juice, or a yoghurt.

Putting
The Metabolic Clock
meal plans
into action

You can create your own weekly meal plans or use the following, which have all the hard work done for you. Use in conjunction with a 21-Day Lifestyle Challenge. The spreadsheets are available at www.metabolicclock.com.

How to use the weekly meal plans

- Use in conjunction with the 21-Day Lifestyle Challenge.

- Allow time on shopping day to sort and prepare your meals for the week. Do a preparation list and prepare some meals. This will make it easy to stay focused on your meal plan as your week gets busy.

- The weekly meal plans are a guide and the ingredients and quantities may vary according to your tastes.

- Some of the midday meal items are easy to buy at cafes if you are out, so you do not have to make everything. These are Thai beef salad, chicken and salmon sandwiches and also meal salads. Japanese restaurants can supply the miso soup, sushi and California rolls.

- Cook extra chicken at meals to have the next day in a meal salad or in sandwiches and mountain bread wraps.

- If you are doing a lot of exercise you can add ¼ cup basmati rice or quinoa to your evening meal or midday meal.

- Experiment with the recipes. If you do not like an ingredient take it out and add something that you do like.

- When compiling your shopping list, check your pantry and refrigerator for the ingredients that you already have.

- The portions used in the recipes may need to be adjusted to suit your energy requirements.

- Make extra of some of the meals. These can be frozen for convenience. Remember that you have them stored and defrost when you know you have a busy day ahead.

- Marinate your meats on shopping day. Freeze the meats to be used later that week. The meats marinate on their way to being frozen and also while defrosting. Remember to defrost the meat in the morning you are going to use it.

Warm weather menu plans for 21-day lifestyle challenge

MENU PLAN WEEK I—WARM WEATHER

SUNDAY

Morning juice—Pineapple, celery, green apple

Breakfast—Poached eggs with wholegrain toast

Mid-morning fruit—2 peaches

Midday meal—Mountain bread wrap of chicken, eggplant dip and salad

Mid-afternoon snack—10 mixed nuts and 1 fig

Evening meal—Stir-fried beef and vegetables, piece of chocolate

MONDAY

Morning juice—Green apple, celery, carrot, ginger

Breakfast—Bircher muesli with mixed berries

Mid-morning fruit—2 slices pineapple

Midday meal—Salmon and salad sandwich on wholegrain bread

Mid-afternoon snack—Seaweed crackers and eggplant dip

Evening meal—Lamb cutlets with ratatouille and salad, chocolate soy ice-cream

TUESDAY

Morning juice—Beetroot, carrot, celery, ginger, green apple

Breakfast—Wholegrain toast with avocado, lemon juice and cracked pepper

Mid-morning fruit—1 nectarine and 1 peach

Midday meal—Pea and spinach frittata with ratatouille salad

Mid-afternoon snack—Vegetable slices with eggplant dip

Evening meal—Lean steak with mixed bean salad, piece of chocolate

WEDNESDAY

Morning juice—Green apple, celery, carrot, ginger

Breakfast—Bircher muesli with mixed berries

Mid-morning fruit—2 slices pineapple

Midday meal—Nutty quinoa salad

Mid-afternoon snack—California roll and green barley juice

Evening meal—Poached salmon with gherkin salsa, chocolate soy ice-cream with nuts

THURSDAY

Morning juice—Pineapple, celery, green apple

Breakfast—Wholegrain toast with tahini and honey

Mid-morning fruit—10 fresh cherries

Midday meal—Niçoise salad

Mid-afternoon snack—10 mixed nuts and 1 fig

Evening meal—Lemon roast chicken, pumpkin, green vegetables, piece of chocolate

FRIDAY

Morning juice—Green apple, celery, carrot, ginger

Breakfast—Bircher muesli with mixed berries

Mid-morning fruit—2 slices pineapple

Midday meal—Mountain bread wrap of chicken, goat's milk feta, eggplant dip, cucumber and lettuce

Mid-afternoon snack—Sushi and green barley drink

Evening meal—Roasted tofu and salad of green beans, butter beans, currents and walnuts, piece of liquorice

SATURDAY

Morning juice—Beetroot, green apple, celery, ginger

Breakfast—French toast with tomato and olive salsa

Mid-morning fruit—10 fresh cherries

Midday meal—Thai beef salad

Mid-afternoon snack—Baked ricotta cake

Evening meal—Curried chicken with warm lentil salad

MENU PLAN WEEK 2—WARM WEATHER

SUNDAY

Morning juice—Pineapple, celery, green apple

Breakfast—Sautéed field mushrooms with wilted spinach and goat's milk feta

Mid-morning fruit—2 nectarines

Midday meal—Thai beef salad

Mid-afternoon snack—Plain rice crackers with beetroot dip

Evening meal—Chicken and vegetable bake with salad, chocolate soy ice-cream with nuts

MONDAY

Morning juice—Green apple, celery, carrot, ginger

Breakfast—Bircher muesli with mixed berries

Mid-morning fruit — Honeydew melon and strawberries

Midday meal—Dhal with kidney beans and chapatti bread

Mid-afternoon snack—10 mixed nuts and 1 fig

Evening meal—Beef with oyster sauce, piece of chocolate

TUESDAY

Morning juice—Beetroot, carrot, celery, ginger, green apple

Breakfast—Smoked salmon and avocado on wholegrain toast with lemon and cracked pepper

Mid-morning fruit—2 peaches

Midday meal—Dhal with kidney beans and chapatti bread

Mid-afternoon snack—Vegetable sticks with beetroot dip

Evening meal—Steak with salad of roasted beetroot, spinach leaves, pistachios, goat's feta, piece of liquorice

WEDNESDAY

Morning juice—Green apple, celery, carrot, ginger

Breakfast—Bircher muesli with mixed berries

Mid-morning fruit — Honeydew melon and strawberries

Midday meal—Nutty quinoa salad

Mid-afternoon snack—California roll and green barley juice

Evening meal—Fish fillets with roasted pumpkin and salad, chocolate soy ice-cream with nuts

THURSDAY

Morning juice—Pineapple, celery, green apple

Breakfast—Poached eggs on wholegrain toast with tomato slices

Mid-morning fruit—1 nectarine and 1 peach

Midday meal—Meal salad with a small can tuna

Mid-afternoon snack—10 mixed nuts and 1 fig

Evening meal—Tuscan chicken and mixed salad, piece of chocolate

FRIDAY

Morning juice—Green apple, celery, carrot, ginger

Breakfast—Bircher muesli with mixed berries

Mid-morning fruit—3 apricots

Midday meal—Quinoa and chicken salad

Mid-afternoon snack—Sushi and green barley drink

Evening meal—Lamb and beans with feta and olive salsa, piece of liquorice

SATURDAY

Morning juice—Beetroot, green apple, celery, ginger

Breakfast—French toast with tomato and olive salsa

Mid-morning fruit—2 slices pineapple

Midday meal—Quinoa and chicken salad

Mid-afternoon snack—Muesli bar

Evening meal—Poached salmon salad with gherkin salsa

MENU PLAN WEEK 3—WARM WEATHER

SUNDAY

Morning juice—Pineapple, celery, green apple

Breakfast—Hard-boiled eggs with wholegrain toast slices

Mid-morning fruit—Mixed berries and natural yoghurt

Midday meal—Meal salad with small can tuna

Mid-afternoon snack—Plain rice crackers with hummus dip

Evening meal—Vegetable stuffed red capsicums and salad, piece of chocolate

MONDAY

Morning juice—Green apple, celery, carrot, ginger

Breakfast—Bircher muesli with mixed berries

Mid-morning fruit—2 slices pineapple

Midday meal—Vegetable stuffed red capsicums and salad

Mid-afternoon snack—10 mixed nuts and 1 fig

Evening meal—Warm meatball salad with hummus, chocolate soy ice-cream with nuts

TUESDAY

Morning juice—Beetroot, carrot, celery, ginger, green apple

Breakfast—Ricotta cheese with fruit spread on wholegrain toast

Mid-morning fruit—2 peaches with 10 raspberries

Midday meal—Niçoise salad

Mid-afternoon snack—Vegetable sticks with hummus dip

Evening meal—Lamb steak with mixed salad and roasted pumpkin, piece of chocolate

WEDNESDAY

Morning juice—Green apple, celery, carrot, ginger

Breakfast—Bircher muesli with mixed berries

Mid-morning fruit—2 slices pineapple

Midday meal—Chicken and salad sandwich on wholegrain bread

Mid-afternoon snack—California roll

Evening meal—Beef with oyster sauce, chocolate soy ice-cream with nuts

THURSDAY

Morning juice—Pineapple, celery, green apple

Breakfast—Ricotta cheese with fruit spread on wholegrain toast

Mid-morning fruit—Small bunch grapes

Midday meal—Mountain bread wrap of hummus, roasted pumpkin and salad

Mid-afternoon snack—10 mixed nuts and 1 fig

Evening meal—Baked salmon steak with salad of grated beetroot, carrot, radish and chopped walnuts, piece of liquorice

FRIDAY

Morning juice—Green apple, celery, carrot, ginger

Breakfast—Bircher muesli with mixed berries

Mid-morning fruit—3 apricots

Midday meal—Mountain bread wrap of chicken and salad

Mid-afternoon snack—Sushi and barley green drink

Evening meal—Lamb and beans with feta and olive salsa, piece of liquorice

SATURDAY

Morning juice—Beetroot, green apple, celery, ginger

Breakfast—Poached eggs with mushrooms and tomatoes

Mid-morning fruit—Small bunch grapes

Midday meal—Thai beef salad

Mid-afternoon snack—Flourless chocolate cake

Evening meal— Orange and ginger chicken with Asian coleslaw

Cold weather menu plans for 21-day lifestyle challenge

MENU PLAN WEEK 1—COLD WEATHER

SUNDAY

Morning juice—Pineapple, celery, green apple

Breakfast—Poached eggs with wholegrain toast, rocket and fresh tomato slices

Mid-morning fruit—2 mandarins

Midday meal—Vegetable soup with pesto and wholegrain roll

Mid-afternoon snack—Flourless orange cake

Evening meal—Chicken and vegetable bake with salad, chocolate soy ice-cream with nuts

MONDAY

Morning juice—Green apple, celery, carrot, ginger

Breakfast—Muesli with poached pears and yoghurt

Mid-morning fruit—2 slices pineapple

Midday meal—Vegetable soup with pesto and wholegrain roll

Mid-afternoon snack—10 mixed nuts and 1 fig

Evening meal—Lamb cutlets with ratatouille and salad, chocolate soy ice-cream

TUESDAY

Morning juice—Beetroot, carrot, celery, ginger, green apple

Breakfast—Baked beans on wholegrain toast

Mid-morning fruit—2 mandarins

Midday meal—Pea and spinach frittata with ratatouille salad

Mid-afternoon snack—Sushi and miso soup

Evening meal—Lean steak with mixed bean salad, piece of chocolate

WEDNESDAY

Morning juice—Green apple, celery, carrot, ginger

Breakfast—Muesli with poached pears and yoghurt

Mid-morning fruit—2 slices pineapple

Midday meal—Nutty quinoa salad

Mid-afternoon snack—California roll and green barley juice

Evening meal—Poached salmon with gherkin salsa, chocolate soy ice-cream with nuts

THURSDAY

Morning juice—Pineapple, celery, green apple

Breakfast—Baked beans on wholegrain toast

Mid-morning fruit—2 kiwifruit

Midday meal—Niçoise salad

Mid-afternoon snack—Protein drink

Evening meal—Lemon roast chicken, pumpkin, green vegetables, piece of chocolate

FRIDAY

Morning juice—Green apple, celery, carrot, ginger

Breakfast—Porridge with maple syrup and milk

Mid-morning fruit—2 slices pineapple

Midday meal—Mountain bread wrap of lemon chicken, goat's milk feta, roasted pumpkin and salad

Mid-afternoon snack—Sushi and miso soup

Evening meal—Fillet of fish with rocket and salad of grated beetroot, carrot, radish and chopped walnuts, piece of liquorice

SATURDAY

Morning juice—Beetroot, green apple, celery, ginger

Breakfast—Wholegrain toast with smoked salmon, avocado, lemon and cracked pepper

Mid-morning fruit—1 pear and 4 walnuts

Midday meal—Thai beef salad

Mid-afternoon snack—10 mixed nuts and 1 fig

Evening meal—Curried chicken with warm lentil salad and steamed green vegetables, piece of chocolate

MENU PLAN WEEK 2—COLD WEATHER

SUNDAY

Morning juice—Pineapple, celery, green apple

Breakfast—Poached eggs with smoked salmon

Mid-morning fruit—2 mandarins

Midday meal—Chicken soup and wholegrain roll

Mid-afternoon snack—Plain rice crackers with beetroot dip

Evening meal—Osso buco with steamed green vegetables, piece of liquorice

MONDAY

Morning juice—Green apple, celery, carrot, ginger

Breakfast—Bircher muesli with kiwifruit and passionfruit

Mid-morning fruit—2 slices pineapple

Midday meal—Chicken and salad sandwich on wholegrain bread

Mid-afternoon snack—10 mixed nuts and 1 fig

Evening meal — Stir-fry beef, ½ cup cooked quinoa, chocolate soy ice-cream with nuts

TUESDAY

Morning juice—Beetroot, carrot, celery, ginger, green apple

Breakfast—Smoked salmon and avocado on wholegrain toast with lemon and cracked pepper

Mid-morning fruit—1 pear, 4 walnuts

Midday meal—Chicken soup with wholegrain roll

Mid-afternoon snack—Vegetable sticks with beetroot dip

Evening meal—Lean steak with mixed salad and roasted pumpkin, piece of chocolate

WEDNESDAY

Morning juice—Green apple, celery, carrot, ginger

Breakfast—Bircher muesli with kiwifruit and passionfruit

Mid-morning fruit—2 slices pineapple

Midday meal—Nutty quinoa salad

Mid-afternoon snack—California roll and miso soup

Evening meal—Fish fillets with roasted pumpkin and salad

THURSDAY

Morning juice—Pineapple, celery, green apple

Breakfast—Porridge with maple syrup and milk

Mid-morning fruit—1 pear, 4 walnuts

Midday meal—Meal salad with a small can tuna

Mid-afternoon snack—10 mixed nuts and 1 fig

Evening meal—Tuscan chicken and salad, piece of chocolate

FRIDAY

Morning juice—Green apple, celery, carrot, ginger

Breakfast—Bircher muesli with kiwifruit and passionfruit

Mid-morning fruit—2 mandarins

Midday meal—Mountain bread wrap of chicken and salad

Mid-afternoon snack—Sushi and green barley drink

Evening meal—Lamb and beans with feta and olive salsa, piece of liquorice

SATURDAY

Morning juice—Beetroot, green apple, celery, ginger

Breakfast—French toast with tomato and olive salsa

Mid-morning fruit—2 slices pineapple

Midday meal—Thai beef salad

Mid-afternoon snack—Muesli bar

Evening meal—Poached salmon salad with gherkin salsa

MENU PLAN WEEK 3—COLD WEATHER

SUNDAY

Morning juice—Pineapple, celery, green apple

Breakfast—Hard boiled eggs with wholegrain toast slices

Mid-morning fruit—1 pear and 4 walnuts

Midday meal—Mountain bread wrap of chicken and salad

Mid-afternoon snack—Flourless chocolate cake

Evening meal—Vegetable and bean soup with pesto and a wholegrain roll

MONDAY

Morning juice—Green apple, celery, carrot, ginger

Breakfast—Baked apple and rhubarb with muesli and yoghurt

Mid-morning fruit—2 slices pineapple

Midday meal—Vegetable and bean soup with pesto and a wholegrain roll

Mid-afternoon snack—California roll and barley green drink

Evening meal—Osso buco with steamed green vegetables, piece of liquorice

TUESDAY

Morning juice—Beetroot, carrot, celery, ginger, green apple

Breakfast—Wholegrain toast with goat's milk feta, pesto and fresh tomato slices

Mid-morning fruit—1 kiwifruit, 1 pear

Midday meal—Osso buco and green salad

Mid-afternoon snack—Vegetable sticks with seaweed rice crackers and goat's milk feta

Evening meal—Vegetable and bean soup with pesto and wholegrain roll, piece of chocolate

WEDNESDAY

Morning juice—Green apple, celery, carrot, ginger

Breakfast—Baked apple and rhubarb with muesli and yoghurt

Mid-morning fruit—2 mandarins

Midday meal—Chicken and salad sandwich on wholegrain bread

Mid-afternoon snack—10 mixed nuts and 1 fig

Evening meal—Herb encrusted salmon, steamed green vegetables, chocolate soy ice-cream with nuts

THURSDAY

Morning juice—Pineapple, celery, green apple

Breakfast—Wholegrain toast with goat's milk feta, pesto and fresh tomato slices

Mid-morning fruit—2 slices pineapple

Midday meal—Meal salad with small can tuna

Mid-afternoon snack—Protein drink

Evening meal—Orange and ginger chicken with steamed vegetables, piece of chocolate

FRIDAY

Morning juice—Green apple, celery, carrot, ginger

Breakfast—Porridge with maple syrup and milk

Mid-morning fruit—1 pear, 1 kiwifruit

Midday meal—Mountain bread wrap of roasted pumpkin, capsicum, goat feta and salad

Mid-afternoon snack—Sushi and miso soup

Evening meal—Lamb and beans with feta and olive salsa, piece of liquorice

SATURDAY

Morning juice—Beetroot, green apple, celery, ginger

Breakfast—Sautéed field mushrooms with wilted spinach and goat's milk feta

Mid-morning fruit—2 slices pineapple

Midday meal—Pea and spinach frittata with rocket, pear slices, walnuts and goat's milk feta

Mid-afternoon snack—Flourless chocolate cake

Evening meal—Warm meatball and pesto salad

A simple formula for sustainable weight loss

The Metabolic Clock will give you a balanced routine and a lifetime of good health.
If you are not burning body fat on this lifestyle then ask yourself the following questions:
 • How many carbohydrates am I having at night?
 • Can I minimise the portions in my meals and stop eating before I feel full?
 • Am I eating breakfast early in the morning?
 • What time am I having my evening meal?
 • Am I eating snack food after my evening meal?
 • Am I skipping meals?
 • What time am I going to bed?
 • Am I chewing my food thoroughly before swallowing?
 • Am I sitting down to eat and relaxing during meal times?

Once you reach your ideal weight you may find that it fluctuates slightly depending upon the amount of carbohydrates you eat and when you eat them. It will become a simple formula for balancing your weight. If you begin to eat more carbohydrates you may notice that you put on body fat. As you notice this, begin to reduce the carbohydrates that you are eating at night. Other ways to bring your body weight into balance are:
 • Adjust your meal portion sizes. If you are not losing weight then you haven't got the right balance for you. Begin to reduce your portions until your comfortable body weight is achieved.
 • Eat a protein and enzyme rich meal in the early evening and don't eat again before going to sleep.
 • Increase the amount of aerobic exercise.
 • Focus on quality sleep. Be in bed before 10 pm and get up early.
 • Stop eating high GI foods that quickly raise your blood sugar level.
 • Focus on re-setting your natural body clock.

You will begin to understand how wonderfully your body responds to being balanced and you'll quickly notice when it is out of balance.

The Metabolic Clock wrap-up

Congratulations on working your way through *The Metabolic Clock* program and beginning your own journey towards balance, good health and wellbeing. At times it can be hard to keep focus and stay committed to a lifestyle program as it is only human to sometimes revert back to old habits, particularly during stressful or challenging times. Here is a list of points to help you keep on track if you ever feel like you might have stumbled slightly. Always go back to the basics to rebalance your metabolic clock.

1. Create compelling reasons and wellness goals to change your lifestyle.
2. Create a daily routine to balance all activities in your day and align your metabolic clock with nature's rhythms.
3. Implement the six daily practices that will bring your digestive system back into balance.
4. See your doctor and have the tests for your Fitness Safety Check. Book times in your diary to begin moving your body.
5. Make the decision to get rid of or minimise foods that are harming you. Implement the five key food choices that will nourish and energise.
6. Take responsibility for your thinking and use the following motivation strategies.
   • Do a mind sweep to sweep out disempowering thoughts and create empowering thoughts.
   • Start to use the three intervention strategies and begin to change bad habits.
   • Create supporting beliefs and make a decision to drop unsupporting beliefs.
   • Visualize your success every day.
7. Start to use chunking to simplify tasks. Make a clean out your cupboards list.
8. Create a 21-Day Lifestyle Challenge to gain momentum.
9. Get your kitchen organized. Start creating weekly meal plans and weekly shopping lists.

For information about Metabolic Clock Programs and free PDF downloads of planning forms visit **www.metabolicclock.com**

Bibliography

Books

Lust John B. 1959, *Raw Juice Therapy*, The Pitman Press, United Kingdom

Meyerowitz, Steve 1984, *Juice Fasting and Detoxification*, Sproutman Publications, United States

Farquharson Marie 1999 *Natural Detox,* Element Books Limited, United Kingdom

Brand Miller Jennie, Foster-Powell Kaye, Colagiuri Stephen, Leeds Anthony 1996, *The G.I. Factor: The Glucose Revolution*, Hodder Headline, Australia

Perricone Nicholas 2004, *The Perricone Promise*, Time-Warner Book Group, United States

Chopra Deepak 1990, *Perfect Health*, Bantam Books, United Kingdom

Lipski Elizabeth 1996, *Digestive Wellness,* Keats Publishing, United States

D'Adamo Peter 2001, *Live Right 4 Your Type*, Penguin Books, Australia

Lad Vasant 1999, *The Complete Book Of Ayurvedic Home Remedies*, Harmony Books, United Kingdom

Urs Koch Manfred 1981, *Laugh With Health*, Renaissance & New Age Creations, Australia

Journals

Chan JL, et al. Ghrelin levels are not regulated by recombinant leptin administration and/or three days of fasting in healthy subjects. J Clin Endocrinol Metab. 2004 Jan;89(1):335-43.

Epel ES, McEwen B, Seeman T, Matthews K, Castellazzo G, Brownell KD, Bell J, Ickovics JR., 'Stress and body shape: stress-induced cortisol secretion is consistently greater among women with central fat.', *Psychosom Med.* 2000 Sep-Oct;62(5):623-32

Di Marzo V, et al. Leptin-regulated endocannabinoids are involved in maintaining food intake. Nature. 2001 Apr 12;410(6830):822-5

Spiegel, K, Tasali, E, Penev, P and Van Cauter E. 2004, 'Sleep Curtailment in Healthy Young Men is Associated with Decreased Leptin Levels, Elevated Ghrelin Levels, and Increased Hunger and Appetite', *American College of Physicians*, 2004; 141 (11), pp846-851.

Tschop M, Weyer C, Tataranni PA, Devanarayan V, Ravussin E, Heiman ML., 'Circulating ghrelin levels are decreased in human obesity.', Diabetes. 2001 Apr;50(4):707

Wang MY, Orci L, Ravazzola M, Unger RH. 'Fat storage in adipocytes requires inactivation of leptin's paracrine activity: implications for treatment of human obesity', *Proc Natl Acad* Sci USA. 2005 Dec13;102(50):18011-16. Epub 2005 Dec 2.

Wren AM, Seal LJ, Cohen MA, Brynes AE, et al., 'Ghrelin enhances appetite and increases food intake in humans.', *J Clin Endocrinol Metab.* 2001 Dec; 86(12):5992.

Press releases

'Running slows the aging clock, Stanford researches find', Stanford School of Medicine Press Release, 11 August 2008

Index

A

acai berry juice 58
action plan 11, 81
additives 41
alcohol 41, 51, 52, 66, 74
ayurvedic 95

B

bacteria 35, 40–1
balance 21–2
    importance of 8, 9, 11, 18
barley powder, green 59
belief 76–8
body image 70–1
bread 102
breakfast 26, 33, 89, 106

C

candida 41
carbohydrates 10, 19, 26, 29, 30, 55, 89
chewing 30, 35, 89
chunking 82–3
circadian rhythms 8, 17
coffee 24, 32, 33, 41, 51–2
colon 35, 36, 38, 41
cortisol 17
creating yourself 67
creative energy cycle 27, 32–3

D

daily routine 22, 33
detoxification 43–4
dieting 8, 10, 18
digestive system 17, 19, 26
    revitalising 35
dinner 134
dips 98–100
disempowering thoughts 68–9, 71–2
drinks
    cleansing 26, 33
    soft 51–2

E

eating out 159
eating slowly 35
emotional eating 8, 11, 25, 62, 66, 73
emotions 64–5, 70
empowered thinking 68, 70–2, 79
energising energy cycle 27, 29
energy 9, 11
    cycles 26

management plan 22
    patterns 24
enzymes 28, 39–40
exercise 8, 33, 45, 89
    afternoon 29
    efficient 48
    emotions and 46
    fun, for 47
    morning 28, 33
    motivation 11
    time, booking 50

F

fats 10
    essential fatty acids 56
fibre 30, 38, 54
    supplement 39, 59
fish oil 59
fitness safety check 50
5-minute rule 73–4, 87
flavour 94–5
    enhancers 96
flour, white 51, 52
food choices 53
fruit 28, 54–5, 58, 89, 116

G

ghrelin 19
glycaemic index (GI) 55
green barley powder 59

H

healthy thinking 62–3
herbs
    dried 95
    fresh 95
hormones 17, 48
    sleep and 19, 26, 31

I

immune system *see* lymphatic system
impassioned thinking 64–7

K

kitchen, organising your 11, 81, 90
    cleaning out cupboards 84–5
    equipment 94
    metabolic clock pantry 91
    strategies 90–1

L

lentils 52
leptin 19
life force 58

lifestyle choices 8, 9, 11, 21
  compelling reasons, creating 13, 88, 169
  nourishing 58
lunch 28, 118
lymphatic system 17, 39, 45

M
marinades 96, 161
'me time' 25
medication 41
meditation 28, 33, 58
melatonin 17, 31
metabolic clock 17, 169
  action plan 11
  balancing 21
  basic principles 89
  cycles 26
  dieting and 18
  getting in tune 22
  what is 18
metabolising energy cycle 27, 28
metabolism 17
  aligning with nature's cycles 17–18
  slowing down 18, 29
  speeding up 8, 11, 13, 48
mind sweep 68, 70–1, 79, 169
momentum
  energy cycle 26–8
  gaining 87
motivation 11, 61, 76

N
nature's cycles 17–18
nervous system 17
nourishment strategies 51

O
oils 56
  fish 59
opinions 66–7
  changing your 68
organic food 52

P
patience 16
pH levels 54
Pilates 28, 33, 45, 47
Pilates, Joseph 45
planning and preparation 83, 94
plant food 35, 41, 54–5
preservatives 41
probiotics 58
processed foods 38, 39, 51, 56, 89

procrastination 24, 77, 81, 82, 85
protein 26, 29, 30, 33, 53, 131

R
raw food 28, 30, 39, 40–1, 52, 54
reading 28
recipes see recipe index
rejuvenating energy cycle 27, 31–2
relaxation 36, 74
  strategies 37
relaxing energy cycle 27, 29–30
reshaping your body 48
responding not reacting 74
rosemary flavour bag 96
running 48–9

S
self-discovery 8
sequencing 83
serotonin 17, 26
shift in perception 66–7
shiftworkers 20
shopping lists 92, 161
sleep 17–18, 33, 89
  'before midnight' 31
  dreamless 32
  importance of 19
  metabolic clock and 19
  tips 32
soft drink (soda) 51–2
sorting 83
spice mix 95
spirulina 59
stress 35, 41, 74
  digestion and 36
success, planning for 82–3
sunrise 20, 26, 32
sunset 20, 29

T
tea 24, 32, 33, 41, 152
  herbal 55
thought viruses 73
thoughts 64, 89
  disempowering 68–9, 71–2
  empowered 68, 70–2, 79
  healthy 62–3
  impassioned 64–7
  unhealthy patterns 73
toxins 26, 43, 45
treats 57, 152
21-Day Lifestyle Challenge 11, 86–8, 169
  cold weather menu plans 165–7
  warm weather menu plans 162–4

U
unhealthy patterns
    changing 74–5
    thoughts 73

V
variety, importance of 95
vegetables 30, 54–5, 100
visualising success 79

W
walking 27, 29, 33, 37, 44, 45, 47, 48, 58, 74,
    83, 87
water 41–3
weekly meal planner 93
    cold weather menu plans 165–7
    using 91, 161
    warm weather menu plans 162–4
weight
    gain 8
    loss 8–9, 43, 59, 168
weight training 28, 48
wellness goals 11, 14–15, 61, 87
    compelling reasons 13–14, 88, 169
    creating 14

Y
yoga 28, 33, 47, 74

Recipe Index

A
apple
    baked, with dates, nuts and yoghurt 115
    baked rhubarb with yoghurt, muesli and 115

B
beans
    dhal with kidney beans 122
    homemade baked 114
    lamb with feta and olive salsa and 148
    soup with pesto 118
    spicy stew 146
beef
    oyster sauce, with 142
    stir-fried 150
    Thai salad 128
beetroot dip 100
berries, fresh
    honeyed yoghurt with almonds and 154
bread 102
    French toast with herb, tomato and olive
        salsa 112
    mountain bread wraps 120
    toppings for toast 114
breakfast ideas 106

C
cake
    baked ricotta 156
    flourless chocolate 152
    flourless orange 154
capsicum
    roasted 100
cheese
    baked ricotta cake 156
    lamb and beans with feta and olive salsa 148
    sautéed mushrooms with wilted spinach and
        goat's feta 112
chicken
    curried, with warm lentil salad 142
    lemon roast with salad 140
    orange and ginger, with Asian coleslaw 150
    quinoa salad and 124
    sandwich 126
    soup with wholegrain bread 120
    Tuscan, with green salad 143
    vegetable bake 143
chickpeas
    hummus 98
chocolate
    flourless cake 152
coleslaw, Asian 150

D

dates
    baked apples with nuts and
    muesli bars with 154
dhal with kidney beans 122
dips 98–100

E

eggplant
    dip 98
    ratatouille 138
eggs
    hard-boiled with wholegrain toast 109
    Niçoise salad 130
    poached 110
    poached with spinach and salmon slices
        110
    tomato and olive open-faced omelette 109

F

fish
    fillets with roasted pumpkin and green
        vegetables 147
    poached eggs with spinach and salmon
        slices 110
    sardines (or mackerel) on wholegrain
        bread 122
    tuna sandwich 126
flavour enhancers 96
French toast with herb, tomato and olive
    salsa 112
frittata, pea and spinach 126
fruit 116 see also by name of fruit

G

ginger and orange chicken with Asian
    coleslaw 150
gremolata 144–5

H

herb, pecan and pistachio crusted, with
    steamed green vegetables 139
herbs
    dried 95
    fresh 95
homemade baked beans on wholegrain
    toast 114
hummus 98

I

ice-cream (soy) with chopped nuts 158

J

juice, morning 104

L

lamb
    beans with feta and olive salsa and 148
    cutlets with ratatouille and salad 138
lemon roast chicken with salad 140

M

mackerel on wholegrain bread 122
marinades 96
meat see also beef, chicken, lamb
    cold with salad 140
    lean, and 4 + 1 salad 136
    osso buco with gremolata 144–5
    warm meatball and pesto salad 140
minted yoghurt dip 98
mountain bread wraps 120
muesli 108
    baked rhubarb and apple with yoghurt and 115
    bars with dates 154
    bircher 108
    poached pears and yoghurt with 106
mushrooms
    pesto field 120
    sautéed with wilted spinach and goat's
        cheese 112

N

Niçoise salad 130
nuts
    baked apples with dates and 115
    herb, pecan and pistachio crusted salmon with
        steamed green vegetables 139
    honeyed yoghurt with fresh berries and
        almonds 154
    pesto 98
    quinoa salad 124
    soy ice-cream with 158

O

olives
    herb and tomato salsa 112
    salsa with lamb and beans 148
    tomato open-faced omelette 109
omelette, tomato and olive 109
orange
    flourless cake 154
    ginger chicken with Asian coleslaw 150
osso buco with gremolata 144–5

P

pasta
    wholemeal or spelt, with fresh tomato and
        basil sauce 128
pea and spinach frittata and salad 126